Self-Care
Deficit Theory
of Nursing

Concepts and Applications

Self-Care Deficit Theory of Nursing

Concepts and Applications

CONNIE M. DENNIS, PHD, RN

Associate Professor, School of Nursing
Illinois Wesleyan University
Bloomington, Illinois

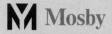 Mosby

St. Louis Baltimore Boston Carlsbad Chicago Naples New York Philadelphia Portland
London Madrid Mexico City Singapore Sydney Tokyo Toronto Wiesbaden

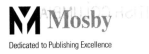
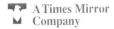

Dedicated to Publishing Excellence

A Times Mirror
Company

Vice President and Publisher: Nancy L. Coon
Editor: Loren S. Wilson
Developmental Editor: Brian Dennison
Project Manager: Linda McKinley
Production Editor: René Spencer
Editing and Production: Top Graphics
Designer: Elizabeth Fett
Manufacturing Manager: Linda Ierardi

Copyright © 1997 by Mosby–Year Book, Inc.

Printed in the United States of America
Composition by Top Graphics
Printing/binding by R.R. Donnelley & Sons

Mosby–Year Book, Inc.
11830 Westline Industrial Drive
St. Louis, Missouri 63146

Library of Congress Cataloging in Publication Data

Dennis, Connie M.
    Self-care deficit theory of nursing: concepts and applications/
Connie M. Dennis.
      p.   cm.
    Includes bibliographical references and index.
    ISBN 0-8151-2426-0
    1. Nursing—Philosophy.   2. Self-care, Health.   I. Title.
    [DNLM: 1. Nursing Theory.   2. Self Care.   WY 86 D411 1997]
RT84.5.D46   1997
610.73'01—dc20
DNLM/DLC
for Library of Congress   96-34177
                                           CIP

97 98 99 00 01 / 9 8 7 6 5 4 3 2 1

*This book is dedicated to my family
who always tried so hard to understand the hours
Mom spent at the computer*

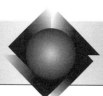

The origins of *Self-Care Deficit Theory of Nursing: Concepts and Applications* go back to 1980, when the faculty of the School of Nursing at Illinois Wesleyan University collectively decided to use Dorothea E. Orem's self-care deficit theory of nursing as the guiding conceptual framework for curriculum and course development. As a member of the first faculty team who taught students in this new curriculum, I helped devise handouts and materials to help guide student learning and practice. Since 1987 I have introduced beginning students to the constructs, concepts, terminology, and other elements of self-care deficit theory of nursing and have provided illustrations of its use in practice. Based on student responses, I worked on developing materials that would simplify student learning and enhance their abilities to generate practice applications in the remainder of the coursework. The materials evolved over the years into the materials compiled in this text.

Purpose

The major purpose of *Self-Care Deficit Theory of Nursing: Concepts and Applications* is to introduce, examine, and interpret Orem's self-care deficit theory of nursing to describe practical applications in nursing practice. First, the material presents a basic introduction to Orem's self-care deficit theory of nursing. At this introductory level the book seeks to provide clear, cogent explication of the constructs, concepts, terminology, and other elements of self-care deficit theory of nursing. Clear definitions with illustrative examples facilitate understanding of the concepts and terms, moving from the abstract level of theory to the more concrete level of practice. Further explication of the theory involves exploration of the relationships between concepts as posed by the three constituent theories of self-care/dependent care, self-care deficit, and nursing system. Second, examples and cases guide and facilitate learning of the self-care deficit theory of nursing by illustrating and applying the principal elements of the theory to practice situations. Examination and analysis of Orem's conceptualizations of nursing and nursing process serve as the groundwork for identification of applications in nursing practice situations. This text evidences a strong nursing focus by emphasizing the use and understanding of the theory for its practical application in patient care situations from health promotion and primary prevention to acute care and long-term care in secondary and tertiary health care situations.

Throughout this book examples and illustrations help to define and illustrate the concepts clearly and to explicate the relationship between these concepts. In addition, the text includes numerous exercises that actively engage the reader in developing an understanding of self-care deficit theory of nursing and Orem's conceptualization of nursing process.

Organization

The organization of the book first introduces the reader to the elements of the theory and, finally, to the application of the theory to patient cases. Chapter 1 introduces the term *nursing theory* and briefly examines the relationship between nursing theory and nursing practice. Statements illustrate the benefits of using Orem's self-care deficit theory of nursing. Chapter 2 presents a general summary of Orem's self-care deficit theory of nursing. An overview of the three constituent theories of self-care/dependent care, self-care deficit, and nursing system introduces major concepts and describes the relationships between the concepts discussed in further detail in subsequent chapters. Chapter 3 focuses discussion on two foundational concepts: deliberate action and basic conditioning factors. These concepts are foundational because they are essential to understanding other concepts in the theory. Deliberate action, as a concept, is essential to understanding action that is self-care/dependent care and action that is nursing. Basic conditioning factors are relevant to both patient variables, therapeutic self-care demand and self-care agency, and the nursing variable, nursing agency. Chapter 4 provides a detailed discussion of the concepts related to the patient variables: (1) therapeutic self-care demand for both self-care and dependent care and (2) self-care/dependent care agency. Chapter 5 presents a discussion of the remaining concepts of self-care deficit theory of nursing. The concepts discussed in this chapter are important to nursing as a helping service: nurse agent, nursing agency, nursing system, nursing situation, and methods of helping.

The remaining chapters of the book focus on explications about Orem's conceptualization about nursing as a practice discipline. Chapter 6 presents an overview of the process of nursing, focusing on the social, interpersonal, and professional-technologic dimensions of nursing practice. The remainder of this chapter focuses on the nursing process, which is the professional-technologic dimension. Discussion of each of the three steps of the nursing process illustrates nursing actions and activities that incorporate the self-care deficit theory of nursing concepts and their relationships. Finally, Chapter 7 presents three case studies for the reader to further explore under-standing of the concepts of the theory and practice activities associated with each of the three steps of the nursing process.

• • •

The intent of this book is purely to introduce the reader to Dorothea E. Orem's work. There is no intention to present a substitute for the original works of Orem. I heartily recommend that readers further explore the depth and richness of this theory by reading Orem DE: *Nursing: Concepts of Practice,* fifth edition, which details most fully and comprehensively the com-plexities of this general theory of nursing.

Connie M. Dennis

ACKNOWLEDGMENTS

Over the years of curriculum development, revision, and refinement, many individuals participated in the discussions of this theory and contributed to the interpretations and resolutions about practice applications. I would like to acknowledge the invaluable input of my colleagues at Illinois Wesleyan University School of Nursing. Many faculty had to sit through long meetings and workshops to discuss how this theory would look in practical application so that we could have concrete examples in the classroom and realistic application in care settings. Many faculty colleagues, especially Donna Hartweg, Sheila Jesek-Hale, and Sharie Metcalfe, were invaluable as "experts," having used this theory in doctoral study and dissertations. Other faculty colleagues, including Margo Tennis, Eileen Fowles, Debra Finfgeld, Jane Brue, Kathy Scherck, and Charla Renner, were eager to help students and, as a result, provided many opportunities for dialogue. Of course, students were often the most critical respondents about whether or not we succeeded in our educational efforts by using this theory of nursing. Therefore I extend a special acknowledgment to the students at Wesleyan who wanted so much to know and understand nursing that they provided the stimulus and motivation for this work. I also thank the manuscript reviewers for their thoughtful suggestions: Sr. Marita Callahan, SP, EdD; Paula E. Frank, RN, PhD; and Effie S. Hanchett, RN, PhD. Last, I would also like to acknowledge the wonderful colleagues and discussions afforded through national and international conferences on self-care deficit theory of nursing, especially those sponsored through the efforts of the University of Missouri-Columbia and the International Orem Society (IOS).

Connie M. Dennis

CONTENTS

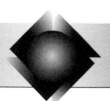

Self-Care Deficit Theory of Nursing

Concepts and Applications

CHAPTER 1

Why Use a Nursing Theory?

KEY TERM

Nursing theory

The purpose of this book is to examine and interpret Dorothea Orem's self-care deficit theory of nursing (SCDTN) to describe practical applications in nursing situations. The discussion that follows is a very brief overview intended to look at the relationship between nursing theory and nursing practice. This approach is particularly important because nursing is a practice discipline.

What Is Nursing Theory?

Nursing theory is a set of concepts and propositions derived from philosophical beliefs about the phenomena of interest to the discipline; relationships between concepts and propositions of a nursing theory purport to describe and explain characteristic phenomena of interest to nursing (Firlit, 1994, p. 76; Marriner-Tomey, 1994, pp. 3–4). Keck (1994) stated that theories serve the purpose of organizing "facts about phenomena of interest to the discipline that comprise the knowledge germane to the discipline" (p. 18). The knowledge about phenomena is organized via propositions, presuppositions, and definitions of concepts and their relationships. The result is a theory. Theory provides a way to organize ideas and concepts so that we can understand, explain, and predict in relation to the events and elements of a discipline (Keck, 1994; Nicholl, 1992). Orem (1995) stated a theory for a practice discipline like nursing is "descriptively explanatory of the dominant features and relationships that characterized the field's practice situations" (p. 167).

Marriner-Tomey (1994, p. 5) described the three "ranges" of theory, defining range as a measure of (1) the breadth and depth of the subject matter addressed by the theory, (2) the scope of the subject matter included in the theory, and (3) the level of abstractness of the formulated theory. These three ranges are grand theory, middle range theory, and micro theory. Grand theory is more abstract, more likely to be all-inclusive, and more complex in that it may often subsume smaller range theories. Micro theory is the least abstract, more narrow and more specific. Middle range theory falls between the two. Marriner-Tomey (1994) defined a conceptual model as "made up of abstract and general ideas (concepts) and propositions that specify their relationships" (p. 4) and then suggested that conceptual models and grand theories are synonymous. Writings of Marriner-Tomey (1994), Nicholl (1992), and Meleis (1991) identified Orem's theory of nursing as a grand theory or conceptual model.

Theory serves a variety of purposes. Historically, nursing theory largely sought to establish nursing as a discipline and promote autonomy of the profession (Blegen & Tripp-Reimer, 1994). Nursing theory provides clarification about how and why nursing is distinct from other health-related professions. Theory serves to organize and categorize and evidence logical systems of thinking about the phenomena of interest to nursing. Theory provides an organizing framework for what is currently known (i.e., current knowledge). Research is a "diligent systematic inquiry or investigation to validate and refine existing knowledge and generate new knowledge" (Burns & Grove, 1993, p. 16). Blegen and Tripp-Reimer (1994) emphasized that a major link between theory and research is between what is known and not known. Nicholl (1992) suggested that a clear purpose of theory is to "provide meaning to the nursing experience" and that the structure of theory provides a frame of reference for nursing decisions (p. 461). Conant (1992) emphasized the contribution of theory to nursing practice stating that theory provides concepts and principles to "guide practice." In this way nursing practice reflects the application of theory. Firlit (1994) and Conant (1992) emphasized that nursing practice contributes to nursing theory in that practice generates questions for further development or research and tests and validates concepts and principles posed by nursing theory. In summary, a nursing theory provides the framework that links nursing research, nursing practice, and nursing knowledge (Figure 1).

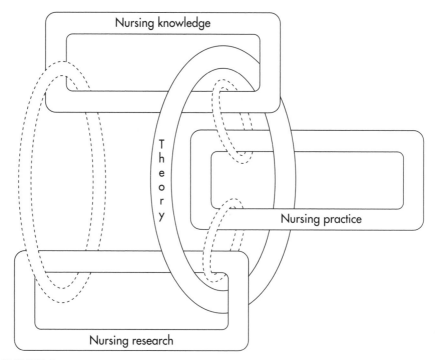

FIGURE 1

Nursing theory provides the link between what nurses know and what nurses do by guiding and directing the selection and use of knowledge. Dotted lines indicate other direct links.

Why Use Orem's Self-Care Deficit Theory of Nursing?

Orem (1995) proposed that a general theory of nursing is an account of the entities and relationships that serve to organize the outlook of nurses (p. 169). Premises about the roles of persons in caring for themselves or others within the context of environment and social groups provide positive views about the maturity and responsibility of the individual and society. It provides a positive frame of reference about nurses, patients, and the interactions between the two. Use of this theory is beneficial in the following ways:

- It promotes a clear understanding of the nature and scope of nursing, especially clarifying what is nursing, what is not nursing, and what nursing could be (Orem, 1995, p. 11).
- It provides direction to nursing practice and nursing research (Orem, 1995, p. 11).
- It maintains a focus on what is relevant to nursing (Orem, 1995, p. 11).
- It provides a common language about nursing to facilitate communication of and about nursing.
- It provides a structure for the endeavors and activities of nurses in nursing situations (Orem, 1995, p. 12).
- It provides a view of commonalities or differences of nursing situations.
- It links relevant knowledge to the requisites of those persons truly in need of the human health–related service that is nursing.
- It provides clarity to the nature of the relationship between nurse and the consumer of nursing: the nurse's patient.
- It specifies outcomes or goals for nursing that facilitate ways in which to demonstrate the effectiveness of nursing care and accountability for nursing actions.

Summary

The concepts and relationships of Orem's self-care deficit theory of nursing (SCDTN) are abstract representations of the real phenomena. The remainder of this text seeks to provide clarifications of the concepts and their relationships and identify applications for nursing situations with patients, particularly through application of a nursing process.

CHAPTER 2

Overview of Orem's Self-Care Deficit Theory of Nursing

OUTLINE

Supporting Background

Theory of Self-Care/Dependent Care

Theory of Self-Care Deficit

Theory of Nursing System

KEY TERMS

Basic conditioning factors (BCFs)

Dependent care

Dependent care agency (DCA)

Dependent care system

Nursing agency

Nursing system

Self-care

Self-care agency (SCA)

Self-care deficit (SCD)

Self-care requisites (SCRs)

Self-care system

Therapeutic self-care demand (TSCD)

Self-care deficit theory of nursing (SCDTN) is the general theory of nursing developed by Dorothea Orem. Self-care deficit theory of nursing is actually the articulation of three theories (Orem, 1995, pp. 170-178). These three theories are the theory of self-care/dependent care, the theory of self-care deficit, and the theory of nursing system (see Figure 2). Because these three theories collectively constitute this general theory of nursing, each of the three theories is a constituent theory of the general theory of nursing. Major theoretical concepts and relationships among these concepts are evident from the constituent theories.

Supporting Background

Various thoughts and conditions provide a basis for the development of this general theory of nursing. Most of these focus on beliefs about the characteristics of persons as human beings (Orem, 1995, p. 169):

- In caring for themselves in their daily lives, persons act deliberately in response to inputs from their internal and external environments. Action made deliberately in response to these inputs is necessary to assure life and well-being and to sustain functional and developmental integrity.
- A person's powers or abilities to respond by acting deliberately is agency. Abilities to act are learned and developed and vary with levels of maturation. Abilities when exercised, or put into action, result in actions that seek to identify and meet the needs of self or others. Therefore action is an expression of the exercise of agency.
- Throughout their lives, persons experience times when they lack the abilities necessary for identifying needs and responding appropriately for themselves or others.
- Exercise of the abilities constituting agency focuses on discovering, developing, and transmitting to self and others ways of acting deliberately to identify and meet requisites of self and others.
- Persons live, grow, and mature within social groups. Group structure and relationships define the roles and tasks of the members. These may vary from culture to culture. Despite variations, common to all social groups is the provision for members who, for varied reasons, may be unable to care for themselves and are dependent on other members of the social group.

The remainder of this chapter is a discussion of each of the three constituent theories in the general theory of self-care deficit theory of nursing. The theory of self-care/dependent care is central to the other two theories and rests at the core of the general theory of nursing. As the core of this general theory of nursing, the theory of self-care/dependent care seeks to provide explanations about persons and how and why they care for themselves or those who are dependent on them. Subsuming this core theory, the theory of self-care deficit seeks to provide explanations regarding persons who have a real need for nursing care. Last, the theory of nursing system subsumes both the first two theories and seeks to describe what is nursing and what is the nature of nursing as helping profession. Figure 2 depicts the relationships and open articulations of these three theories.

Theory of Self-Care/Dependent Care

The theory of self-care/dependent care (Orem, 1995, pp. 171-174) is the first of the three constituent theories. It represents the core of the general theory of self-care deficit theory of nursing because it focuses on two major concepts: self-care and dependent care. Understanding of other essential concepts evident in this theory is dependent on the core concepts of self-care and dependent care. Other concepts include self-care requisites, therapeutic self-care demand, self-care and dependent care agency, and basic conditioning factors. The next chapter focuses on the definitions and relationships of these concepts; this section discusses the framework provided by the theory of self-care/dependent care. Concepts are evident in the discussion of the nursing theory.

Logical antecedent statements of beliefs serve as presuppositions (Orem, 1995, pp. 171-172). As presuppositions, these statements establish necessary

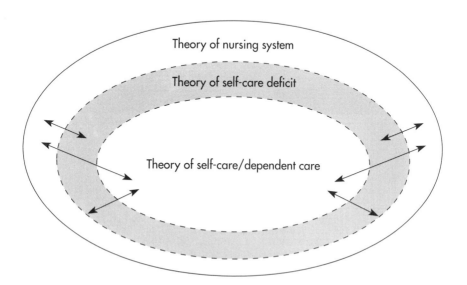

FIGURE 2

Three interrelated theories in the framework of Orem's self-care deficit theory of nursing (SCDTN).

conditions on which the nursing theory builds its general principles. These include the following:

- Mature and maturing persons employ both intellectual and psychomotor skills to provide daily care for themselves (self-care) or for those dependent on them (dependent care). Care actions are continuous and require maintenance of the drive and motivation to provide self-care (or dependent care) on a continuing, daily basis. Varying degrees of effectiveness in achieving self-care (or dependent care) result from the person's actions.
- Accomplishment of self-care or dependent care requires actions that procure, secure, and use various resources.
- Within the context of social and cultural groups, persons learn valid actions to meet the requisites for self-care (or dependent care). Variations in life situations and social context create different circumstances that affect the selection or desirability of responsive actions or action repertoires.
- Persons establish patterns of action (action repertoires), often establishing set patterns of behaving based on past successes and personal preferences. These patterns of action affect or demonstrate whether persons act toward self-care or not. Some behaviors become so routinized that they constitute habits for self-care (dependent care).
- The abilities and actions are learned. Learning of and preferences for self-care (or dependent care) actions are largely gained by experience with the need for care and ways to meet it.
- Scientific knowledge or formal systems of information supplement experiential knowledge in determining what requisites should be met and how to meet them.

The central idea posed by the theory of self-care/dependent care emphasizes that persons perform discrete actions or sequences of actions directed toward themselves or their environment (self-care) or directed toward the care of those dependent on them (dependent care). These actions are self-care actions or dependent care actions, respectively. Persons perform self-care (or dependent care) in the process of daily living and continuously over time (i.e., from day to day to day). The actions and action sequences that constitute self-care (or dependent care) are deliberately performed. A basic assumption is that self-care (or dependent care) actions have purpose and that the purpose is to meet known self-care requisites essential for daily care of self (or others, as in dependent care). Meeting requisites that pertain to self-care (or dependent care) results in the regulation of structural and functional integrity and human development. Actions that are regulatory strive to meet three types of requisites: (1) those *universal* to all persons, (2) those specific to human *developmental* processes, and (3) those associated with *deviations* in a person's state of *health* (health deviation).

The overall goal of all self-care actions is to contribute to one's own life and self-maintenance and to promote one's own personal health and well-being. The overall goal of all dependent care actions is to promote and maintain the life and developmental processes and to promote the health and well-being of the dependent person.

Persons learn self-care actions within the context of their sociocultural/family group throughout the process of development and maturation. Development of dependent care actions also occurs through the learning processes. For example, adults may have early learning experiences of role-modeling and role-playing for parenting skills; they could also engage in formal education such as prenatal classes or college classes related to parenting skills.

Orem made several additional statements that provide more information about the theory of self-care/dependent care and the development of self-care (or dependent care) as a theoretical concept (Orem, 1995, pp. 173-174; 1991, pp. 69-70; 1985, pp. 36-37). The following interdependent and inter-related statements add further clarification to some of the complexities of the theory of self-care/dependent care:

- Self-care requisites (SCRs) express both the need for care and actions for meeting those needs.
  1. There are three categories of self-care requisites: (1) universal self-care requisites (USCRs) are common to all human beings, (2) developmental self-care requisites (DSCRs) are specific to the conditions/events of the related developmental state, and (3) health deviation self-care requisites (HDSCRs) originate from conditions of illness or injury in the health state.
  2. The origin of self-care requisites comes from the individual's internal or external environment and also from the individual's resources and energy available for meeting these self-care requisites.
  3. Basic conditioning factors (BCFs; age, gender, developmental state, health state, health care system, sociocultural orientation, family system, patterns of living, environment, and available resources; see pp. 24-25) influence both the need and action components of self-care requisites. Basic conditioning factors affect all persons.
  4. Knowledge of self-care requisites, including varied ways of meeting self-care requisites, is evident in specific sets of processes or technologies. *Technologies* refers to the knowledge and the intellectual and psychomotor abilities essential to the action.

5. Repetition in dealing with and meeting known, recurring self-care requisites leads to established and known action repertoires (i.e., common, repeated, successful ways of doing or acting) and the formation of habits for self-care.

- Clustering, organizing, and sequencing discrete actions create action systems for self-care or dependent care (i.e., **self-care system** or **dependent care system**).

   1. Actions performed to meet self-care requisites are deliberate forms of action performed with some degree of completeness and effectiveness to meet known requisites for functioning and development. The overall intent is to do good, that is, to contribute positively to the promotion and maintenance of structural, functional, and developmental integrity and the promotion of life and well-being.

   2. The self-care system (or dependent care system) addresses known universal, developmental, and health deviation self-care requisites attending to the interrelationships between and among the self-care requisites. Action systems consist of an organized series of discrete actions. The intent of self-care systems is to meet self-care requisites. The intent of dependent care systems is to meet the self-care requisites of the dependent person.

   3. The self-care system (or dependent care system) results when the person takes action to meet known self-care requisites based on deliberate choices. Operations essential to deliberate action involve (1) intellectual activities related to investigating and delineating what needs to be and what actions will result in this end, (2) intellectual activities related to judging and selecting what course of action is desirable to meet the desired end, and (3) acting on those choices. The final step is the person performing care actions that result in the achievement of self-care (dependent care). A major intent is that the resultant self-care (or dependent care) is of therapeutic quality.

- Persons gain knowledge and abilities about self-care/dependent care.

   1. Knowledge of self-care actions (or dependent care actions) is developed through investigation, observation, and practice.

   2. Self-care actions and dependent care actions are learned within a cultural context. Thus self-care actions (or dependent care actions) may vary with the individual and among larger social groups. All persons have (1) the potential for learning and developing abilities to care for self (or others) and (2) the potential for being motivated to care for self (or others).

Some definitions of terms have been developed in the theory of self-care/dependent care. These terms are important for the discussion of both the theory of self-care deficit and the theory of nursing system. Although these concepts and terms appear in much greater detail later in this book, the following list includes some simple definitions that permit further discussion of the theories:

- **Self-care** is action performed on behalf of one's self to meet one's own self-care requisites.
- **Dependent care** is action performed by one person to meet the self-care requisites of another person. Examples of dependent care are a mother caring for her infant, a son caring for his older adult mother who has a chronic illness, a wife caring for her husband who is a quadriplegic.
- **Self-care requisites (SCRs)** are the needs for self-care and the actions necessary for meeting those needs. Self-care requisites are the purposes or goals of self-care or dependent care.
- **Therapeutic self-care demand (TSCD)** is the totality of all the self-care requisites necessary for achieving therapeutic self-care at one point in time.
- **Self-care agency (SCA)** is the complex set of acquired abilities for carrying out the actions for meeting self-care requisites.
- **Dependent care agency (DCA)** is the complex set of acquired abilities for carrying out actions for meeting self-care requisites of a dependent person.
- **Basic conditioning factors (BCFs)** are conditions or events that characterize the features of the person, the self-care requisites, or the abilities of the person for performing actions.

Theory of Self-Care Deficit

The theory of self-care deficit "expresses and develops the reasons why persons require nursing" care (Orem, 1995, p. 174). To do so, the theory embraces the definitions and characteristics of self-care and dependent care as discussed in the theory of self-care/dependent care. Important aspects of self-care are that self-care (1) requires the ability to engage in self-management continuously over time, (2) is essential to life and well-being and integrity of physical and psychological functioning, and (3) is directed toward meeting known self-care requisites. Factors such as the person's intellectual and psychomotor abilities, valuation of the requisites to be met, maturity, sociocultural-spiritual orientation, and available resources affect both the quality and quantity of self-care (or dependent care).

The following statements about societies and social groups are foundational for understanding the theory of self-care deficit (Orem, 1995, p. 174; 1991, p. 71; 1985, pp. 35-36):

- Societies are made up of individuals living in social groups and units.
- Social groups are the context in which self-care is learned.
- Society provides for dependency of its members, institutionalizing and giving sanction to groups to aid those in need according to the nature of the dependency. The nature of the dependency is a result of age-related factors or other basic conditioning factors.
- The health care services are examples of socially institutionalized groups aimed at helping persons who experience social dependency when the reason for the dependency is health related.
- Nursing is one of the health care services in society.

The central idea of the theory of self-care deficit rests on the tenet that humans are subject to changes in structural, functional, or developmental integrity. Such changes may be health related or health derived and may result in new needs for self-care (or dependent care). Also, changes in the external environment may create new needs for self-care (or dependent care). Change may trigger immediate needs for self-care (or dependent care), whereas anticipation of change facilitates projection of new needs and what these could mean in terms of changes in or adjustments to self-care (or dependent care) actions. New or anticipated needs may be beyond the current developed abilities of the person to engage in self-care actions (or dependent care actions; i.e., self-care agency and dependent care agency, respectively). Resultant limitations in the abilities to carry out or perform self-care actions (or dependent care actions) are self-care limitations. Self-care limitations may inhibit or render the individual completely or partially incapable of producing (1) continuous self-care (or dependent care) *or* (2) self-care (or dependent care) that is effective or adequate in meeting the self-care requisites (Orem, 1995, 1991).

The theory of self-care deficit focuses on the relationship between the therapeutic self-care demand (the total of all self-care requisites) and the self-care (or dependent care) agency (the abilities for meeting the self-care requisites). A **self-care deficit (SCD)** represents a relationship in which the therapeutic self-care demand exceeds self-care agency. If the therapeutic self-care demand of a dependent care recipient exceeds dependent care agency, then dependent care deficit exists. When health-derived or health-related self-care limitations result in deficits and interfere with the production of self-care (or dependent care), persons have self-care (or dependent care) deficits and have a need for nursing. Persons with health-derived and health-related self-care limitations arising from insufficient or unused self-care agency or dependent care agency are of concern to nurses because these persons cannot meet their therapeutic self-care demand and cannot, therefore, accomplish therapeutic self-care (or dependent care). A person whose self-care agency or dependent care agency is equal to or exceeds the therapeutic self-care demand has no need for nursing. Thus the presence of self-care deficits (or dependent care deficits) indicates why a person has a need for nursing care and why the person is a legitimate patient of nursing.

Orem has made a variety of statements that contribute to the development of self-care deficits as a theoretical entity. The following interdependent and interrelated statements aid in the understanding of the theory of self-care deficit (Orem, 1995, pp. 174-175; 1991, pp. 70-71; 1985, pp. 34-36):

- With regard to self-care agency (or dependent care agency):
  1. Persons engaged in self-care (or dependent care) have specialized, learned abilities for action. Self-care agency (SCA; or dependent care agency [DCA]) is the set of human abilities for deliberate and continuous engagement in self-care actions (or dependent care actions). These abilities are learned and developed over time in mature and maturing individuals.
  2. The individual's abilities related to self-care actions (or dependent care actions) are modified or conditioned by basic conditioning factors (age, gender, developmental state, health state, health care system, sociocultural orientation, family system, patterns of living, environment, and available resources).
- With regard to the relationship between self-care requisites and self-care agency (or dependent care agency):
  1. The relationship between the therapeutic self-care demand and self-care agency (or dependent care agency) can be determined only after demand and agency are first assessed. The relationship between the two entities can be expressed in terms of therapeutic self-care demand being equal to, less than, or greater than self-care agency (or dependent care agency).
  2. When therapeutic self-care demand is greater than self-care agency (or dependent care agency), a deficit relationship exists. This deficit relationship is a self-care deficit (or a dependent care deficit, respectively).
- With regard to the nature of self-care deficits:
  1. When there is a current deficit relationship between the therapeutic self-care demand and the self-care agency, this is an *existing self-care deficit*. When the relationship between the two suggests a foreseeable, predictable deficit relationship, this is a *projected self-care deficit*.
  2. Self-care deficits can be temporary or permanent. With development of skills, knowledge, or motivation in self-care agency, with assistance in mobilizing unused abilities, or with reduction of therapeutic self-care demand, self-care deficits can be overcome. Persisting self-care deficits may indicate a need for dependent care or ongoing helping services.

3. One way to express self-care deficits is as statements of action limitations associated with the operations of deliberate action.
4. The presence of either existing self-care deficits or projected self-care deficits establishes acceptable social dependency that justifies and legitimizes the need for the human helping service of nursing (i.e., the self-care agency of the individual is inadequate to meet the current need or is assessed as being inadequate to meet new or upcoming needs). These statements similarly pertain to dependent care deficits (see Chapter 4).

Theory of Nursing System

The preceding theories describe the nature of self-care and self-care deficits. Persons with health-derived or health-related self-care deficits (or dependent care deficits) are persons who have a need for and can be helped by nursing. The theory of nursing system (Orem, 1995, pp. 175-177; 1991, pp. 72-73; 1985, pp. 37-38) embraces the first two theories and establishes the nature of the helping service provided by nurses in nursing situations. This theory introduces the nursing variable of nursing agency and related concepts. The following statements about nursing are foundational to the understanding of the theory of nursing system:

- Nursing is a helping service sanctioned and institutionalized by society.
- Nursing is complex, deliberate action performed by nurses to assist others.

The central idea of the theory of nursing system focuses on the helping service provided by nurses. A **nursing system** is an action system created and executed by nurses and directed toward those health-derived or health-related self-care deficits (or dependent care deficits) of persons engaged in self-care or dependent care (self-care agent or dependent care agent, respectively). The actions that make up these complex nursing systems are the result of nurses deliberately exercising those specialized, learned abilities for providing nursing (exercise of **nursing agency**). The end goals of all the actions and interactions produced by the nursing system are to (1) protect or develop existing self-care (dependent care) agency or to regulate the exercise or development of self-care agency (or dependent care agency) and (2) assist patients in achieving therapeutic self-care.

Nursing systems occur within interpersonal and contractual relationships. These relationships exist between persons who legitimately occupy the role of nurse and persons who legitimately occupy the role of patient (legitimate patients of nursing). The patient becomes the legitimate concern of nursing when there are existing or projected self-care deficits. Designs of nursing systems aim at overcoming or compensating for the self-care (or dependent care) deficits for individuals (including dependent care units) or multiperson units (Orem, 1995, p. 349). Multiperson units may be a group of persons making up a family, groups of persons with a similar need for self-care or similar self-care limitations, aggregate groups, or communities.

The following interdependent and interrelated statements aid in further understanding the theory of nursing system (Orem, 1995, 1991, 1985):

- All persons have existing and projected self-care requisites. Those persons determined to have existing self-care (dependent care) deficits or projected self-care (dependent care) deficits are legitimate patients of nursing.
- With regard to interactions:
  1. Nurses establish interpersonal interactions with legitimate patients of nursing. The sociointerpersonal relationship is the context in which nursing action is taken.
  2. The combined actions of the nurse and the patient, aimed at assuring that the self-care requisites are met, make up the nursing system. The actions of both are complementary.
- With regard to descriptors of those actions that are part of the nursing endeavor:
  1. Nurses assess the patient's existing and projected self-care requisites, including the identification and selection of valid modes of actions necessary for meeting identified self-care requisites.
  2. Nurses assess the patient's abilities to meet current and anticipated self-care requisites, including the use of known technologies to meet self-care requisites.
  3. Nurses further determine when the patient, for therapeutic reasons, should refrain from performing self-care actions and when the patient must refine current abilities for self-care or develop new abilities for self-care (i.e., make changes in self-care agency).
  4. Nurses determine plans of care that will ensure that necessary steps are taken to meet those self-care requisites therapeutically. Nurses may act to support or develop the patient's self-care agency (dependent care agency) or to reduce the needs for self-care (dependent care).
  5. Nurses and patients always act concertedly to ascribe and allocate roles for the prescription, production, and regulation of therapeutic self-care and in the regulation of the exercise or development of self-care (dependent care) agency.

Summary

Together, the theories of self-care/dependent care, self-care deficit, and nursing system constitute the total framework of self-care deficit theory of nursing (SCDTN). A major assumption basic to self-care deficit theory of nursing is: Persons perform actions that when directed to their own needs for care (or the care of dependent others) produce action systems known as self-care (or dependent care) (Figure 3). Nurses use the theory's structural framework and knowledge of the concepts and their relationships to one another in practice to do the following:

- Determine the patient's total demand for self-care (therapeutic self-care demand).
- Ascertain the patient's abilities for engaging in self-care (self-care agency) or abilities for engaging in dependent care (dependent care agency).
- Determine the influence of basic conditioning factors that modify or condition both the self-care demand and the self-care (dependent care) agency.
- Identify the relationship between the patient's therapeutic self-care demand and current self-care agency (i.e., identifying if either existing self-care deficits or projected self-care deficits exist).
- Determine what aspects of self-care (or dependent care) can be or should be managed by the patient or the patient's support system and design an appropriate action system for nursing care to address these aspects (nursing system).
- Plan and initiate methods by which the nurse can best help the patient or the patient's support system.
- Judge the success of the designed nursing system or the need for continuance or modification of the nursing system.

Nurses develop knowledge and abilities for engaging in nursing actions (i.e., nursing agency) through nursing education and experience. Through the exercise of nursing agency, nurses identify persons with self-care (dependent care) deficits, provide appropriate help via designed nursing systems, and evaluate the outcomes of nursing care. Use of nursing theory to guide the intellectual processes of investigation, interpretation, judging, critical thinking, and problem-solving assists nurses in developing nursing agency and in providing the kind and type of nursing care needed by patients.

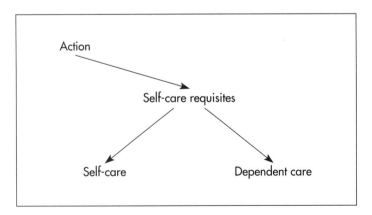

FIGURE 3
Actions directed toward self-care requisites produce self-care (dependent care).

E X E R C I S E

Basic Definitions

In the development of every nursing theory, a "language" also develops. This language consists of the terms or phrases that represent primary and secondary concepts expressed within the theory. Use of and versatility in the language of a nursing theory helps nurses to better communicate ideas consistently. The preceding discussion introduced important terms of self-care deficit theory of nursing. Begin to build your vocabulary of theoretical terminology. For each of the following, provide a brief definition and, if appropriate, include the acronyms.

1. Self-care _____

_____

_____

_____

2. Dependent care _____

_____

_____

_____

3. Basic conditioning factors _____

_____

_____

_____

4. Self-care requisites _____

Universal _____

_____

Developmental _____

_____

Health deviation _____

_____

5. Therapeutic self-care demand _____

_____

_____

_____

continued

6. Self-care agency _____

_____

_____

_____

7. Dependent care agency _____

_____

_____

_____

8. Self-care deficit _____

    Existing _____

    _____

    Projected _____

    _____

9. Nursing system_____

_____

_____

_____

10. Nursing agency _____

_____

_____

_____

Examining Foundational Concepts

The focus of this chapter is to address two foundational concepts: deliberate action and basic conditioning factors. The two main concepts presented are foundational since they provide essential background necessary for understanding other concepts in self-care deficit theory of nursing (SCDTN). The concept of deliberate action permeates self-care actions, dependent care actions, and nursing actions. The concept of basic conditioning factors is the foundation of understanding all about persons, in particular, those persons engaged in self-care or dependent care (i.e., self-care agents or dependent care agents) and those persons engaged in providing nursing care (i.e., nursing agents). Basic conditioning factors, when looked at in terms of person aggregates, can provide a helpful analysis of the nature of the aggregate.

Deliberate Action

Exploration of the concept of deliberate action is an appropriate starting point because both self-care and nursing care are types of deliberate action in Orem's self-care deficit theory of nursing. Understanding the concept of deliberate action is a crucial part of understanding the nature of self-care and nursing care. A major assumption underlying this concept is that persons are capable of rational thought and exercising reason. Aspects of human development and maturation involve learning how to engage in deliberate action.

Orem (1995) defined **deliberate action** as "action to achieve a foreseen result that is preceded by investigation, reflection, and judgment to appraise the situation and by a thoughtful, deliberate choice of what should be done" (p. 229). Emphasis is placed on persons thinking before they act and that goal-oriented action follows decision. As such, deliberate action is clearly different from instinctual acting or from physiological response.

Addressing two questions will help to better understand this concept: What constitutes action? and What makes action deliberate? Performing or doing something (mental or physical) over time constitutes an action. Actions, often thought of as single entities, are really several sequential, individual acts. For example, "getting dressed" is an action undertaken most every morning. Yet getting dressed may involve several acts such as putting on undergarments followed by putting on slacks, sweater, socks, and shoes. Putting on slacks, a chosen action, consists of several discrete acts: holding slacks in readiness before standing on the right leg while inserting the left leg, then standing on the left leg while inserting the right leg into the correct slack leg, pulling the pants up over the hips, fastening the button at the waist, and then pulling up the zipper. Even the act of pulling up the zipper consists of a series of organized, sequential acts. Tying a shoelace is another example. When watching a 4-year-old learning to tie a shoelace, one can readily see the individual acts necessary to accomplish the action. Yet, for most adults, tying shoes is a single act that, in turn, is part of the larger action of putting on their shoes. Sequencing of actions to achieve a desired result may vary from one situation to another. For example, one might put the left leg into the slacks first at one time or at another time put the right leg into the slacks first. Some changes in action sequences do not alter the achievement of the desired result. Some changes in action sequences will alter the outcome. An example of this latter statement is putting on one's pants before putting on one's undergarments. The previous discussion illustrates that actions (1) may be simple, compound, or complex and (2) occur in a logically ordered sequence to achieve a desired result.

Deliberate action is action resulting from investigative, reflective, and productive processes. Employing the processes of investigation and reflection, persons identify what must be accomplished and why. Processes of reflecting and judging facilitate making decisions about what to do based on existing factors, conditions, and personal values. Productive, reflective, and investigative processes are necessary to initiate and take action in accord with the decision made and to determine whether the chosen action, once performed, achieves the desired expected outcome.

Phases of Deliberate Action

The actions that make up deliberate action occur in two distinct phases: the intentional phase and the productive phase (Orem, 1995, pp. 115-116). Each phase has associated sets of operations. An **operation** is an intellectual or psychomotor action directed toward a goal or end result. **Sets of operations** refer to clusters of related operations (i.e., actions) that may or may not be sequential and that delineate the ways and means of achieving a specific result.

Intentional Phase. The first phase of deliberate action is primarily intellectual. Actions of this phase center on gathering or processing information about what is and what should be. This phase, the intentional phase, has two sets of operations: the estimative and the transitional (Orem, 1995, pp. 230-232). **Estimative operations** are those investigative and reflective actions in which the individual explores, examines, analyzes, and contemplates the nature of the situation, including relevant factors intrinsic and extrinsic to the individual. The person comes to understand the situation, including how it is currently and/or how it could or should be. Knowledge is a key element for this phase; this includes knowledge from scientific sources as well as from common sense. The end result of estimative operations is to know what is, what could be or should be, and alternatives on how to achieve what could or should be. In self-care these estimative operations contribute to identification and prescription of what self-care actions are needed and why. In nursing care estimative operations contribute to the formulation of a nursing diagnosis (i.e., what nursing is needed and why).

Transitional operations are those judging and decision-making actions in which the course of action is decided. Actions associated with transitional operations focus on determining which outcome(s) and action(s) are valued over others. The end result is a decision about what outcome is good and desired and a decision about what action or actions will contribute to meeting the expected outcome. In self-care this operation focuses on choosing from various alternatives about what to accomplish and what to do to accomplish it. These decisions contribute to formulations of plans about what will be the person's plan for self-care. In nursing these operations also contribute to formulations about the plan for nursing care.

An important point in this first phase of deliberate action is that most actions are intellectual. Although primarily intellectual, some psychomotor actions are useful for collecting and gathering information (e.g., going to the library or health department for information sources). Because one cannot make decisions on what is not known, estimative operations must precede transitional operations.

Productive Phase. The second phase is one of producing action. In this, the productive phase, energies and efforts focus on carrying out selected actions to meet the desired, expected outcome. Analysis of actual outcomes in contrast to the desired outcomes is another critical process of the productive phase. Analysis leads to judgments about whether to continue, substitute, or alter the action plan. A unique set of operations occurs in the productive phase: productive operations (Orem, 1995, pp. 232-234). **Productive operations** include all the psychomotor activities related to carrying out the action(s), as well as those activities that help to ascertain whether actions result in the desired, expected outcomes. Planning, organizing, and coordinating are activities that are clearly important. Another important action includes evaluating, at appropriate points, to determine the status of the desired, expected outcome. Initiating actions and persevering in acting are crucial to achieving outcomes. One must employ both cognitive and motor abilities. Other factors that influence the achievement of desired, expected outcomes are motivation, commitment, energy, and physical dexterity and movement. The end result of the actions making up the set of productive operations is the actual production and accomplishment of an action system. In Orem's self-care deficit theory of nursing, the action systems produced are self-care, dependent care, or nursing care. In self-care, self-care actions are produced. In nursing, nursing actions are produced.

In this second phase of deliberate action, the actions are primarily psychomotor. Processes focus on carrying out actions as planned to meet the desired, expected outcomes. At times, input of new data or change in factors will necessitate modifications in the actions being produced. The intellectual component of this phase includes analysis of new or different input and information about the actions as performed or about the desired, expected outcomes. This phase consists of actions manifested in the behavior of the person. Because it consists of behavior, the productive phase of deliberate action is the most easily observed and measured.

The nature of deliberate action is to appraise a situation and to take specific action(s) for achieving desired, expected outcomes. In general, deliberate action is analogous to what individuals do in any problem-solving situation: (1) they examine the problem and identify known alternative solutions or approaches to the problem, (2) they critically analyze the alternative approaches to the problem and the anticipated outcome(s) of each, (3) they decide on a plan of action, (4) they then act on that decision by carrying out the action, and (5) finally, they determine if the outcome was the one desired and expected.

The two phases of deliberate action, intentional and productive, emphasize the significance of both intellectual processes and manipulative processes. Action is not random. Rather, action follows careful consideration and decision-making about what should be accomplished (i.e., the desired, expected outcome) and the ways and means (i.e., actions) of achieving the outcome. Deliberate action is not an instinctual response; nor is it a response made reflexively. Knowledge, motivation, desirability, and commitment are key factors in determining the desired, expected outcome and in delineating the actions necessary to achieve that outcome (Figure 4).

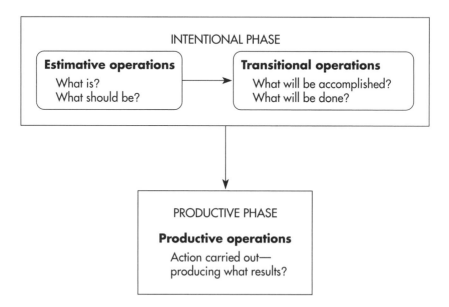

FIGURE 4
Phases of deliberate action.

Basic Conditioning Factors

Basic conditioning factors (BCFs) (Orem, 1995, pp. 203-204, 284-288) are those characteristic attributes, properties, or events internal or external to the person that make each individual and his or her self-care requisites unique. A factor, as defined by Orem, is a constituent element that actively contributes to or exerts influence or effect on a complex whole thing (Orem, 1995, p. 82). Factors are basic in that they are fundamental and apply to all persons. Factors are conditioning in that they actively influence or modify a person's need for self-care or dependent care and a person's abilities for action. Orem described 10 factors as conditioning; these factors are discussed later in this section.

For persons engaged in self-care (i.e., self-care agents or dependent care agents), basic conditioning factors directly or indirectly influence the need for self-care (self-care requisites) and the desired, expected outcomes associated with meeting these self-care requisites. Thus basic conditioning factors modify or effect *self-care requisites,* collectively known as therapeutic self-care demand. This also means that basic conditioning factors influence or effect, directly or indirectly, the person's abilities for performing self-care (or dependent care), that is, self-care agency (or dependent care agency). The basic conditioning factors characterize the person engaged in self-care or dependent care (the self-care agent or dependent care agent) because they provide insight about qualities and traits that influence the individuality of who and what the person is. When applied to aggregates, the basic conditioning factors help to characterize one aggregate as like or unlike another aggregate.

Basic conditioning factors also characterize persons in the role of nurse. When basic conditioning factors are examined, they help to explain and describe the uniqueness of every nurse. The basic conditioning factors emphasize that nurses are persons with underlying characteristics that influence who they are as a nurse. The same basic conditioning factors are conditioning for the nurse as they are for the self-care agents and the dependent care agent. These basic conditioning factors actively influence the abilities of the nurse to plan and perform nursing care, that is, nursing agency (Figure 5).

The basic conditioning factors identified by Orem (1995, p. 203), as modified by the author, are listed below:

1. Age: Current chronological age
2. Gender: As either male or female
3. Developmental state: The physical, functional, cognitive, and psychosocial level
4. Health state: The current and past health states of the person and the person's own perception of health
5. Health care system: The system in which health care is both accessible and available to the person

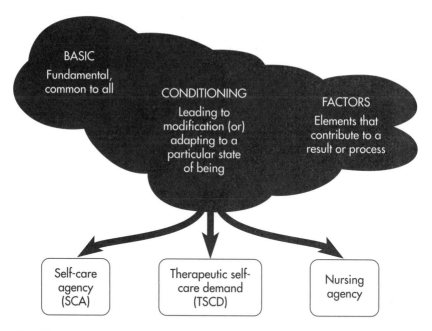

FIGURE 5

Basic conditioning factors modify self-care agency, therapeutic self-care demand, and nursing agency.

6. Sociocultural–spiritual orientation*: The multiple, complex, and interrelated system of the person's social environment and spiritual belief system

7. Family system: The multiple, complex and interrelated system of interpersonal and social relationships and functions of the family unit

8. Patterns of living: The person's usual, normal self-care actions

9. Environment (conditions of living): The environmental setting in which the person normally engages in self-care or dependent care actions

10. Available resources: Resource availability, accessibility, and resource utilization

Table 1 provides further exploration of these 10 basic conditioning factors by suggesting parameters for assessing the status and values of each factor. This is not an all-inclusive list but should give the reader a framework for understanding and exploring each of the basic conditioning factors.

---

*Although Orem does not make specific note of the influence of the factor of spirituality, the author determined that the modifying influence of this factor is noteworthy and substantiated sufficiently to be included herein. The strong link between sociocultural, ethnic, and religious factors are established well enough to include it with the single sociocultural factor.

TABLE 1 Basic Conditioning Factors and Relevant Assessment Data		
Conditioning Factor	**Descriptor**	**Assessment of Data Relevant to Factor**
1. Age	Current chronological age	Determine time elapsed from birth and ascertain age-related modifications of self-care requisites or age at onset of health deviation(s).
2. Gender	As either male or female	Determine if gender-related modifications of self-care requisites exist or if self-care actions alter or vary because of gender.
3. Developmental state	The physical, functional, cognitive, and psychosocial developmental level	Determine if physical growth and developmental task work are appropriate for age (chronological) and for condition (health state). Aspects addressed include developmental milestones and tasks, growth parameters, development of thought processes (e.g., concrete versus abstract, reasoning, problem-solving, reading, thinking, comprehending). Determine the ability to engage in and maintain social relationships.
4. Health state	The current and past health states of the person and the person's own perception of his or her health	Determine the health state before and during the current time via the process of health and medical history (personal and family), general health state (as from a review of systems), current problems or complaints, diagnostic (medical and nursing) and treatment response data. Judge what is perceived as necessary to recover from illness or injury and the responses to current or changed status. Detect the meaning and type of impact health state has on lifestyle.
5. Health care system	The system in which health care is both accessible and available to the person	Determine what measures are instituted in or by what medical/health care institutions (and their relevant policies); what are the roles, actions, and practices of various health care team members; and how these are coordinated. Detect what is the resultant form of care.

TABLE 1 Basic Conditioning Factors and Relevant Assessment Data—cont'd		
Conditioning Factor	**Descriptor**	**Assessment of Data Relevant to Factor**
6.-7. Sociocultural-spiritual orientation/family system*	The multiple, complex, and interrelated system of the person's social environment and spiritual belief system and social relationships and function of the family unit	Determine what the living context is, including language, education, occupation, occupational/life experiences, ethnic-cultural background and practices, health beliefs, religion and practices pertaining to spirituality, place in family constellation, roles/relationships of family members and significant others, impact of health state on family as unit and on family members, and economics of the family. Determine not only what is culturally acceptable but what is culturally prescribed.
8. Patterns of living	The person's usual, normal self-care actions	Determine which self-care actions are performed daily or at other regular intervals, the amount of time devoted to self-care, the person's priority ratings of self-care actions, individual perceptions of adjustments/changes in self-care actions caused by health state, health care system, or actions not related to self-care.
9. Environment (conditions of living)	The environmental setting in which the person normally engages in self-care actions	Determine the person's usual place of residence and conditions under which daily self-care is produced. Aspects addressed about home environment include (space, location, and crowding).
10. Available resources	Resource availability, accessibility, and resource utilization	Determine resources available within and without the person's living environment and which are currently used and which are needed. Resources include economic, personnel, agencies (organizations), and time. Detect perceptions about resource adequacy.

*Because of the close association of sociocultural-spiritual orientation and family system as part of the learning and living context of persons, these two factors are considered together.

Some basic conditioning factors are relatively stable over time. Some factors change rapidly from one point in time to another. For example, age in an adult tends to be more stable as a basic conditioning factor than age in an infant or toddler. Health state is relatively stable in a person in a rehabilitation center when compared with the stability of health state in a trauma patient in an emergency department. The basic conditioning factors characterize the individuality of each person and significantly influence the relationships that persons establish with one another.

Understanding basic conditioning factors is important for persons as they perform self-care or dependent care. Persons engaged in self-care or dependent care (i.e., self-care agents or dependent-care agents) must develop knowledge of the ways in which these factors influence both the requisites for self-care (i.e., collectively, therapeutic self-care demand) and the abilities for meeting self-care or dependent care (i.e., self-care agency or dependent care agency). It is also important that nurses who seek to provide nursing care understand and comprehend the modifying and qualifying effect of these basic conditioning factors. For nurses, two basic reasons substantiate the need for knowledge about basic conditioning factors. First, understanding distinguishing characteristics of persons will enable the nurse to better help and collaborate with meeting and achieving therapeutic self-care. Knowledge of basic conditioning factors may help to predict or explain variations in persons' self-care requisites or variations in persons' abilities to perform care (agency). The basic conditioning factors may also condition the type and amount of assistance persons will accept. Second, nurses must have a good understanding of the ways in which their own basic conditioning factors influence their nursing agency and the nursing care they produce.

Basic conditioning factors are explored and understood in relation to their modifying influence on (1) the value of self-care requisites being met, (2) performing self-care actions to meet self-care requisites, and (3) abilities for taking deliberate action. The exercises at the end of this chapter help to explore this concept.

Summary

Two major concepts explored as foundational are deliberate action and basic conditioning factors. Each is considered foundational in that it affects the understanding of several other concepts in the self-care deficit theory of nursing. The concept of deliberate action affects the understanding of the two major conceptual elements of theory: self-care (and dependent care) and nursing care. Both self-care (and dependent care) and nursing care are forms of deliberate action. The concept of deliberate action emphasizes that self-care systems (and dependent care systems) and nursing systems (1) employ intellectual and psychomotor processes and (2) initiate and sustain action by choice rather than random behavioral or physiological response. The concept of basic conditioning factors emphasizes that internal and external factors influence and characterize persons engaged in self-care and dependent care (self-care agents and dependent care agents) and persons engaged in nursing care (nurse agents). These basic conditioning factors affect the major patient variables of therapeutic self-care demand and self-care agency in that they influence or modify the person's self-care requisites and his or her abilities for meeting those self-care requisites. The conditioning factors affect the major nurse variable (nursing agency) in that they influence or modify the nurses' abilities for engaging in nursing activities. Chapters 4 and 5 further illustrate the relationship of these foundational concepts to other concepts of the theory.

E X E R C I S E

Identifying Basic Conditioning Factors

PART I

In the space at the right of each item below, identify the basic conditioning factors suggested by the data provided in the item on the left. More than one basic conditioning factor is applicable to each item.

Data	*Basic Conditioning Factors*
1. Sixteen-year-old male admitted for diagnostic tests.	Age, gender, health state
2. Father died of myocardial infarction 6 months ago.	
3. Employed part-time in factory line work.	
4. Mennonite farmer admitted for hernia repair.	
5. Father lives with son and family in ranch home and gets a community "mobile meal" for lunch.	

continued

Data	Basic Conditioning Factors
6. Twenty-two-year-old female Jehovah's Witness admitted for labor and delivery.	_____
7. Thirty-seven-year-old coal miner admitted to the intensive care unit for acute respiratory distress.	_____
8. Four-year-old admitted for urinary tract infection; mother concerned about regression in toilet training.	_____
9. Widow, 84 years old, expresses concerns about being admitted to nursing home for the first time.	_____

PART II

For each of the 10 basic conditioning factors, identify at least one piece of information that characterizes you as a self-care agent each day. How does this affect the self-care action or the quality or quantity of the self-care action?

1. Age
_____
_____
_____

2. Gender
_____
_____
_____

3. Developmental state
_____
_____
_____

4. Health state
_____
_____
_____

5. Health care system
_____
_____
_____

6. Sociocultural-spiritual orientation
_____
_____
_____

7. Family system
_____
_____
_____

continued

Data	Basic Conditioning Factors
8. Patterns of living	_____ _____ _____
9. Environment	_____ _____ _____
10. Available resources	_____ _____ _____

EXERCISE

Nurses and Basic Conditioning Factors

PART I

In the space at the right of each item below, identify the basic conditioning factors suggested by the data provided in the item on the left. More than one basic conditioning factor is applicable to each item.

Data	Basic Conditioning Factors
1. Registered nurse holds degree from inner city New York program and grew up and worked in same area.	_____ _____ _____
2. Registered nurse with master's degree in gerontology provides wellness care within community clinic.	_____ _____ _____
3. Registered nurse must juggle part-time work with care of school-aged children and commitments to Lutheran church where she is a member of the lay board.	_____ _____ _____
4. Following a divorce, 49-year-old returns to nursing after working only in her home setting for past 25 years.	_____ _____ _____

continued

Data	Basic Conditioning Factors
5. Filipino nurse passes licensure examinations and completes orientation to new large medical center in Chicago.	_____ _____ _____

PART II

For each of the 10 basic conditioning factors, identify at least one piece of information that characterizes you as a nurse at this point in your nursing career.

1. Age

    _____
    _____
    _____

2. Gender

    _____
    _____
    _____

3. Developmental state

    _____
    _____
    _____

4. Health state

    _____
    _____
    _____

5. Health care system

    _____
    _____
    _____

6. Sociocultural-spiritual orientation

    _____
    _____
    _____

7. Family system

    _____
    _____
    _____

8. Patterns of living

    _____
    _____

9. Environment

    _____
    _____
    _____
    _____

10. Available resources

    _____
    _____
    _____

EXERCISE

Basic Conditioning Factors of Groups/Communities

Basic conditioning factors can be used to describe the characterizing features of groups or communities. Using these factors, one can identify ways in which the group or community is heterogeneous or homogeneous. Use the basic conditioning factors to assess (1) a small group of students in a class, the entire class, or school or (2) a community in which you live.

Key Concepts: Self-Care/Dependent Care and Self-Care Deficit

The focus of this chapter is on key concepts contained within the first two constituent theories of Orem's self-care deficit theory of nursing: the theory of self-care/dependent care and the theory of self-care deficit. The discussion of the foundational concept of deliberate action in the preceding chapter provides insight about the nature of action and action systems. The concept of deliberate action is foundational to the discussion of self-care (or dependent care) and self-care (or dependent care) as an action system (self-care system [dependent care system]). The concepts derived from and related to these two theories include self-care, self-care requisites (universal, developmental, and health deviation), therapeutic self-care demand, self-care agency, and self-care deficits. The definition and interpretation of concepts also culminate in the exploration of relationships among the concepts. To eliminate some confusion, the initial discussion focuses on self-care and the concepts of self-care requisites, therapeutic self-care demand, self-care agency, and self-care deficits. Later, discussion expands to incorporate the concept of dependent care. Comparisons and contrasts between self-care and dependent care help to delineate ways in which dependent care and dependent care systems are like or unlike self-care and self-care systems.

Self-Care

Self-care is the voluntary production and practice of actions directed toward one's self or one's environment to regulate one's own functioning and development and is aimed at maintaining life, health, and well-being (Orem, 1995, p. 95). Self-care, in its totality, consists of all actions deliberately undertaken daily by an individual to care for one's self. These actions are called self-care actions. **Self-care agent** is the term for the person providing self-care (Orem, 1995, p. 104), and the person providing self-care is self. Numerous, often clustered, sequenced self-care actions make up self-care. As such, self-care constitutes an *action system*. In the action system of self-care (called self-care system in this text), all related self-care actions (both simple and complex) are performed in some order when caring for one's self.

Characteristics of Self-Care

Several characteristics of self-care are inherent in the concept. Understanding each of these feature characteristics facilitates further understanding of the full extent and nature of the concept of self-care. Figure 6 illustrates the interrelated characteristics that help to describe self-care. The following discussion focuses on these characteristics.

Self-care is an action system. Multiple, discrete actions within larger action systems make up self-care. The various larger action systems collectively constitute the total self-care system. The action taken is *deliberate* (see discussion of deliberate action in preceding chapter). The major implication about action as deliberate is that knowing precedes deciding, which, in turn,

SELF-CARE

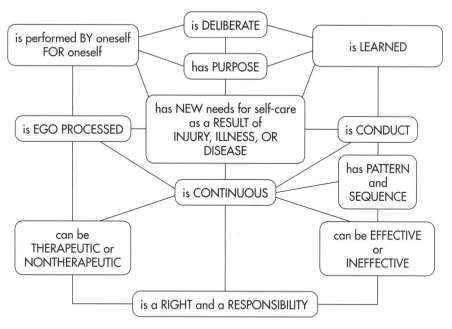

FIGURE 6

The interrelated characteristics of self-care.

precedes acting. As a result, self-care is neither haphazard nor random. Self-care is not instinctual. How to act and behave in order to care for one's self is *learned* over time. The context for learning self-care is one's social and cultural environment. The initial and primary source is the family unit; but as the person's social sphere increases, the sources for learning expand. Behavior is learned throughout the periods of maturation. Importantly, new learning can influence, change, or redirect the current level of self-care for any person.

Inherent in the definition of self-care and in the term itself, self-care is *performed by oneself for oneself* (Orem, 1995, p. 95). This emphasizes that the direction of self-care is always toward self. Actions performed for another, to meet another's self-care requisites, do not constitute self-care. In keeping with this aspect of the concept, self-care is *ego processed*. It is self-oriented, self-directed, and self-produced.

Actions in self-care systems are directed toward the ultimate *purpose* of maintaining one's whole being contributing to the sustenance and maintenance of human structural integrity, human functioning, and human development (Orem, 1995, p. 103). Self-care actions, then, are goal directed with the goals being the self-care requisites (the needs or demand for care). Self-care is action in response to a need or demand for care of one's self. The focus of self-care is always that it constitutes action initiated and performed to care for self to meet known self-care requisites, which are the goals or purposes. Perceptions of self-care as action to meet personal needs for self-care (self-care requisites) emphasize that self-care is personal *conduct.* Physical, emotional, and intellectual maturity affect the behavior or conduct called self-care action. Self-care as conduct also implies that self-care is behavior managed and directed by the person.

Orem stated that self-care is a *continuous* contribution to life, functioning, and well-being. This would strongly suggest that self-care is one of the most basic forms of health care. Performed on a continuing basis, it is essential to maintenance of life. Self-care is not a stop-and-go process. One cannot get up in the morning and just decide that today will be a day free of all self-care actions. Some self-care requisites continue daily on a regular pattern, for example, self-care requisites for managing urine and bowel elimination or maintaining a sufficient intake of air. These self-care requisites, if ignored, lead to serious consequences. Skipping oral hygiene for one day may not lead to serious consequences. Other self-care requisites occur on a recurring pattern, not necessarily a daily pattern. For example, women must manage their menses every cycle. Needs and the actions necessary to meet the needs also change with maturation and development. In instances of illness, injury, or disease, *new needs for self-care* (new or altered self-care requisites) arise. Therefore the needs (or self-care requisites) are everchanging. Regardless, some self-care requisites must be met each day on a continuing basis.

Consistent with the concept of deliberate action, the self-care actions performed by self-care agents are directed toward desired, expected outcomes. Based on accumulated and evergrowing knowledge (both of the scientific kind and the common sense kind), self-care actions are associated with certain expected outcomes. Different self-care actions or self-care action systems may lead to the same expected outcome. Deliberate action involves not only the selection of a desired outcome but also the selection of which actions, of all those possible, will lead to this desired, expected outcome. Achievement of the desired, expected outcome is supportive of the efficacy of the self-care actions. When the actions of the self-care system achieve the desired, expected outcomes, the self-care system is *effective.*

The selected self-care actions or desired outcomes may not always be *therapeutic,* that is, have a positive contribution to life and well-being. Some self-care actions or desired outcomes may indeed be nontherapeutic. Examples of persons acting toward nontherapeutic outcomes or using nontherapeutic actions include the person who smokes one to two packs of cigarettes a day, the person with diabetes who regularly selects and eats foods not part of the prescribed diet, or the person who does not put on a seat belt when driving a car. In these examples, the outcome desired by the person may focus on an alternative expected outcome: for example, smoking to prevent weight gain associated with quitting or to appear more sophisticated and "adult" within the peer group. Although it is desirable that self-care be therapeutic, in reality, not all decisions for self-care lead to positive behaviors or outcomes.

Once actions are initiated to achieve self-care, the performance of self-care actions occurs in a logical sequence of related acts (i.e., the self-care system). Sometimes self-care actions must be carefully articulated with one another to assure achievement of the desired, expected outcome (see discussion of action and action sequences in the preceding chapter). Self-care action, therefore, has *pattern* and *sequence*. Consider the self-care action of brushing one's teeth. The orderly sequence involves putting toothpaste on a toothbrush before brushing and rinsing. Actions are related to one another. One step logically precedes another. To alter the pattern and sequence of a set of self-care actions can lead to poor, inadequate, or alternate outcomes. For example, brushing teeth before eating or putting on socks after shoes will definitely influence desired, expected outcomes. Clustering and sequencing of actions to achieve an outcome results in an action system. The action system of self-care actions for brushing teeth is distinct from the cluster of self-care actions for putting on shoes and socks. The action system of self-care actions for putting toothpaste on a toothbrush is part of the larger action system of self-care actions for brushing one's teeth but is distinct from the self-care actions of actually brushing the teeth with the brush.

Orem stated that self-care is voluntary (Orem, 1995, p. 112). This would suggest that the person may choose to engage in self-care action or not. Yet, societal expectations reinforce the *responsibility* of self-care and acknowledge the right and responsibility of the individual (especially an adult) to make decisions and choices essential in the concept of deliberate action. Societies do define situations of acceptable social dependency and provide means for caring for those who are acceptably dependent on others for care.

Orem suggested that self-care is a *right*. Persons have a rightful claim to care that contributes to promoting and maintaining human structural, functional, and developmental integrity. Such a view emphasizes that others who seek to care for another must legitimate their role in caring for that person, especially justifying how and why that person cannot provide for self.

Self-Care Requisites

Self-care is action directed toward meeting purposeful, expected outcomes. The formulated, expressed purposes toward which self-care actions are directed are known as **self-care requisites (SCRs)** (Orem, 1995, pp. 108–

E X E R C I S E

Characteristics of Self-Care

From the discussion of the concept of self-care, identify the meaning of each of the following characteristics ascribed to self-care. Discuss the implications of each of the characteristics descriptive of self-care.

1. Self-care is PERFORMED by ONESELF for ONESELF.

2. Self-care is EGO PROCESSED.

3. Self-care is DELIBERATE.

4. Self-care is LEARNED.

5. Self-care is CONDUCT.

6. Self-care has PATTERN and SEQUENCE.

7. Self-care has PURPOSE.

8. Self-care has NEW NEEDS (FOR SELF-CARE) as a RESULT of INJURY, ILLNESS, or DISEASE.

9. Self-care is CONTINUOUS.

10. Self-care can be EFFECTIVE or INEFFECTIVE.

11. Self-care can be THERAPEUTIC or NONTHERAPEUTIC.

12. Self-care is a RIGHT and a RESPONSIBILITY.

109). Self-care requisites are generalizations (Orem, 1991, p. 122) about the need for self-care and the ways (actions) of attaining self-care. This statement illustrates that self-care requisites actually have two parts. The first part represents the need which persons must meet to achieve or maintain life, health, integrated functioning, and well-being. The need is the factor or element that is to be controlled or regulated by self-care actions (Orem, 1995, p. 108). The second part emphasizes that specific types, qualities, and quantities of self-care action (Orem, 1995, p. 187) are necessary for meeting the specific need for self-care. This latter emphasis indicates self-care requisites are more than just needs for self-care. Self-care requisites must suggest what self-care actions are necessary to meet the need for self-care. Because this definition of self-care requisites stresses that a "requisite" is both the need and the action to meet the need, *requisite* is a much more accurate term than *need*. However, it is not unusual to interchange the phrases "need for self-care" and "self-care requisites" in common usage.

The basic conditioning factors modify self-care requisites in two ways. First, one or more basic conditioning factors may affect the value, quality, or quantity of the self-care requisite itself. For example, the number of calories or nutrients required daily can vary according to age, gender, or health state. Sociocultural-spiritual orientation can modify the method of food preparation, availability, and consumption. Environment can also modify methods of food preparation and storage. Second, some or all of the basic conditioning factors can modify or specify the technologies required for meeting known self-care requisites. *Technology* is the term used by Orem (1995, pp. 182, 189) to designate the means and methods of accomplishing a purpose, in this case, a self-care requisite. Application of knowledge about the need for self-care and the associated self-care actions is an important aspect of the term *technology*. The following example illustrates how basic conditioning factors affect the technologies for meeting self-care requisites associated with urine or fecal elimination: in an infant a diaper is the method for "controlling" elimination, whereas in an older child or an adult the usual means is self-controlled toileting. Basic conditioning factors relevant in this example are age, developmental state, and health state. Environment and sociocultural-spiritual orientation can modify definitions of toileting practices, for example, some cultures do not diaper the infants.

Orem (1995, pp. 108, 191) described three separate but interrelated categories of self-care requisites:

1. Universal self-care requisites (USCRs)
2. Developmental self-care requisites (DSCRs)
3. Health deviation self-care requisites (HDSCRs)

Each category of self-care requisites contains multiple requisites: (1) the category of universal self-care requisites include eight different requisites, (2) the category of developmental self-care requisites includes two types of requisites, and (3) the category of health deviation self-care requisites includes six types of requisites. A more detailed discussion of each category follows. First, however, a discussion focuses on the concept of particularized self-care requisites.

As stated previously, each self-care requisite is a generalization about the need for and ways of attaining self-care. To understand a specific need for self-care, the requisites must be examined and judged in light of known basic conditioning factors. Orem (1995, pp. 266, 331) stated that basic conditioning factors that must always be considered are age, developmental state, and health state. These basic conditioning factors most actively condition the self-care requisites. When appropriate, inclusion of other basic conditioning factors helps to quantify or qualify either the need for self-care or the self-care actions. **Particularized self-care requisites (PSCRs)** are definitive statements or expressions of self-care requisites formulated to provide specific individual qualifications about the need for self-care and the ways and means (actions) necessary to meet that need. As an action-oriented statement, the particularized self-care requisite specifies the degree and type of actions necessary to meet a self-care requisite for a particular individual at a particular point in time (Orem, 1995, pp. 110-111, 188, 270). More than one particularized self-care requisite may be necessary to address the scope of a self-care requisite fully for an individual. Particularization means that the movement is made from the general self-care requisite to the particular, from the more abstract to the concrete. Consistent with the concept of self-care as deliberate action, persons (nurses and self-care agents) must first know and understand the need for self-care in terms of particular action or sets of sequential action.

The following sections provide a discussion of each of the three categories of self-care requisites. Each section contains examples of particularized self-care requisites to provide clarification through illustration. Following the sections that discuss each category of self-care requisites, a discussion shifts to focus on the process of particularizing self-care requisites (formulating or expressing particularized self-care requisite statements).

Universal Self-Care Requisites

Universal self-care requisites (USCRs) make up the category of self-care requisites that represent the basic needs that must be met to achieve or maintain optimum functioning, health, and well-being (Orem, 1995, pp. 191-196). Universal self-care requisites are common to all humans and are constantly present throughout each stage of the life cycle. The quantity and quality of the needs for self-care and the associated care actions vary in life according to the influence of basic conditioning factors (age, gender, developmental state, health state, health care system, sociocultural-spiritual orientation, family system, patterns of living, environment, and available resources [see pp. 24-25]). Persons act to change, prevent, mitigate, or minimize conditions/events arising from or affecting internal functioning or environment. Universal self-care requisites, when met therapeutically and effectively, contribute to positive support of life processes (physical, cognitive, and emotional), structural and functional integrity, maturation, health, and well-being (Orem, 1995, pp. 108-109).

The following eight types of universal self-care requisites are common to males or females of any age as described by Orem (1995)★:

1. Maintenance of a sufficient intake of **AIR**
2. Maintenance of a sufficient intake of **WATER**
3. Maintenance of a sufficient intake of **FOOD**
4. Provision of care associated with **ELIMINATION** processes and excrements
5. Maintenance of a balance between **ACTIVITY AND REST**
6. Maintenance of a balance between **SOLITUDE AND SOCIAL INTERACTION**

★Words in **boldface** type indicate the factor being regulated or controlled in the self-care requisite toward which self-care actions are directed.

7. **PREVENTION OF HAZARDS** to human life, human functioning, and human well-being
8. Promotion of human functioning and development within social
groups in accord with human potential, known human limitations,
and the human desire to be normal **[NORMALCY]**

The first three universal self-care requisites of air, water, and food focus
on necessary materials and resources that supply these elements that are essential for life and bodily processes. The focus is not only what amounts are
appropriate and safe but also on factors, internal and external, which, when
controlled, contribute to and are life sustaining. Similarly the fourth universal self-care requisite, elimination, focuses on needs for self-care and care
actions associated with the various routes of excrements. These elimination
processes must support life processes. Self-care actions center on support of
the elimination process, control of the waste products, and control of impact
on the environment. The fifth and sixth universal self-care requisites, ac-
tivity/rest and solitude/social interaction, respectively, focus self-care actions on the need for harmonious balance in life between two extremes.
The control of time, degree and amount of activity, and interests pursued
provide energy outlets and promote a sense of well-being. Achievement
of a balance between solitude and social interaction is necessary. The inner
self and self autonomy develop through reflection and contemplation, while
at the same time social relationships, emotional ties, and trust develop with
others. Prevention of hazards focuses on the control the person has over
both internal and external environments. Closely linked with all the other
universal self-care requisites, potential hazards associated with all requisites
must be controlled or monitored to protect and promote human functioning and development. The last universal self-care requisite maintains a close
relationship with each of the other seven. Promotion of normalcy, like prevention of hazards, focuses on control of internal threats with the intent to
develop positive personal attributes such as responsibility, sense of self, and
completeness. Orem's description (1995, p. 193) of general sets of actions associated with each of the universal self-care requisites provides further clarification of each universal self-care requisite (Table 2).

Examples
Each of the eight universal self-care requisites is presented below with an
example of a particularized self-care requisite focusing on that universal
self-care requisite. The action verb in each particularized self-care requisite
statement denotes the general method (i.e., the usual or expected way) of
acting to achieve that goal/purpose of self-care (the self-care requisites).
Further discussion of the general method and particularization of self-care
requisites follows the discussion of the three categories of self-care requi-

TABLE 2 Sets of Actions Associated With Meeting Universal Self-Care Requisites

Factor Focused on in Universal Self-Care Requisite (USCR)	Broad Sets of Action Relevant to Control or Regulation of Factor Focused on in Universal Self-Care Requisite*
Air Water Food	Identify, attend to, and provide amounts or quantities necessary to support of related life processes. Control of external factors that affect availability, quality, and accessibility and control of internal factors that affect consumption. Control of consumption or intake with pleasure and without abuse, thus contributing optimally to integrated functioning. Preserve and protect anatomical structures and physiological processes.
Elimination	Control or regulate internal or external factors that affect the normal function and bodily processes associated with elimination of body products. Manage bodily functions and protect anatomical structures associated with elimination. Dispose of all excrements and waste products (physiological and environmental) safely and wisely. Carry out all personal body hygiene and physical care. Care for and protect environment.
Activity and rest	Select and engage in activities that keep physical movement in balance, stimulate affective responses, promote intellectual efforts, and provide for social interaction. Identify, attend to, control, and regulate factors that promote activity and rest and a balance between the two. Maximize incorporation of personal interests and employment of personal abilities within culturally prescribed norms and personal values when developing, maintaining, or adjusting a pattern of rest and activity.
Solitude and social interaction	Strive for and manage personal, individual autonomy; strive for personal satisfaction and enjoyment in group memberships; strive for a balance between the two. Develop and foster bonded, enduring relationships with others in which (1) mutual love, affection, and friendship are shared experiences and (2) both self and others are mutually considered and served. Demonstrate respect for others' integrity, rights, and individuality. Recognize, control, and regulate factors (internal and external) that affect the quality and balance between actions conducive to reflection in solitude and activities that promote socialization.

Modified with permission from Orem, D. (1995). *Nursing: Concepts of practice* (5th ed., p. 193). St. Louis, MO: Mosby.
*Actions presented here are intended to illustrate and are not intended to be all-inclusive.

continued

TABLE 2 Sets of Actions Associated With Meeting Universal Self-Care Requisites—cont'd	
Factor Focused on in Universal Self-Care Requisite (USCR)	**Broad Sets of Action Relevant to Control or Regulation of Factor Focused on in Universal Self-Care Requisite**
Prevention of hazards	Identify, attend to, control, and regulate hazards that exist or are likely to exist.
	Exercise preventive efforts to avoid or eliminate events or conditions that could prove harmful to physical, mental, or emotional well-being.
Normalcy	Develop and maintain positive perception of self, self-concept, and body image.
	Foster all aspects of human development.
	Identify integrity in human structure and functioning or deviations; act to promote and maintain integrated human functioning and structure.

sites. Words cited in parentheses after the example illustrate basic conditioning factors that modify or influence the value of the self-care action or type of self-care action.

- **AIR:** Breathe 16 to 18 times per minute (adult).
- **WATER:** Drink six to eight 8-oz glasses of water daily (adolescent/adult).
- **FOOD:** Consume a 1500-calorie, balanced diet daily (adult with obesity in health state).
- **ELIMINATION:** Bathe daily (sociocultural-spiritual orientation).
- **ACTIVITY AND REST:** Jog 1 mile daily (adult in good health state). Sleep 8 to 10 hours nightly (child or adult).
- **SOLITUDE AND SOCIAL INTERACTION:** Interact with family members. Spend time alone for at least 1 hour daily.
- **PREVENTION OF HAZARDS:** Avoid foods high in cholesterol.
- **NORMALCY:** Voice perception of self as competent in occupation (adult).

Developmental Self-Care Requisites

Developmental self-care requisites (DSCRs) are those basic needs/goals derived from and associated with human development and the self-care actions to meet those needs (Orem, 1995, pp. 196-200). Developmental self-care requisites have a strong relationship and connection with the universal self-care requisites. Developmental needs (for self-care) are those needs for self-care that pertain to the control or management of conditions or resources necessary to support or promote normal human development

(Orem, 1995, p. 197). In essence, developmental self-care requisites are specialized expressions of universal self-care requisites that have a unique developmental focus or emphasis. Indeed, these were initially part of the universal self-care requisites but were later given separate designation "to emphasize their importance and because of their number and diversity" (Orem, 1995, p. 196). The diversity and scope of theories and knowledge regarding developmental processes is extensive. This contributes to the complexity of understanding the human dimension of development and the self-care actions necessary to meet developmental needs (Orem, 1995, p. 196).

The distinctive focus of developmental self-care requisites is their expression of the requisites associated with developmental stages/phases. Orem (1995, p. 197) stated that the conditions associated with developmental self-care requisites arise from the following stages of the life cycle (Figure 7):

- Fetal, including birth
- Neonatal
- Infancy
- Childhood and adolescence
- Adulthood
- Pregnancy in either adolescence or adulthood

These stages closely approximate the develomental stages associated with various chronological ages. In most developmental texts, however, discussions of childhood and adulthood evidence more stages of development than suggested here. Developmental needs may be associated with growth and physical development, psychosocial and emotional development, cognitive development, or language development. Applying growth and developmental theories, the varying events/conditions associated with each stage of development challenge the individual with various developmental tasks. Individuals must take action to meet the demands posed by the developmental task.

Types of Developmental Self-Care Requisites. Orem described three sets of developmental self-care requisites: provision of conditions that promote development, engagement in self-development, and interferences with development (Orem, 1995, pp. 197-200). The first two sets address conditions that, when met or acted on, will promote development of self. There is one major difference between these two sets. In the first set, persons (usually because of age) are dependent. Others must perform actions on their behalf to meet developmental needs and to promote development. In the second set, persons are actively involved in the processes of development. The third set of developmental self-care requisites focuses on actions necessary to mitigate or prevent interferences from conditions, events, or situations that could have a deleterious effect on development.

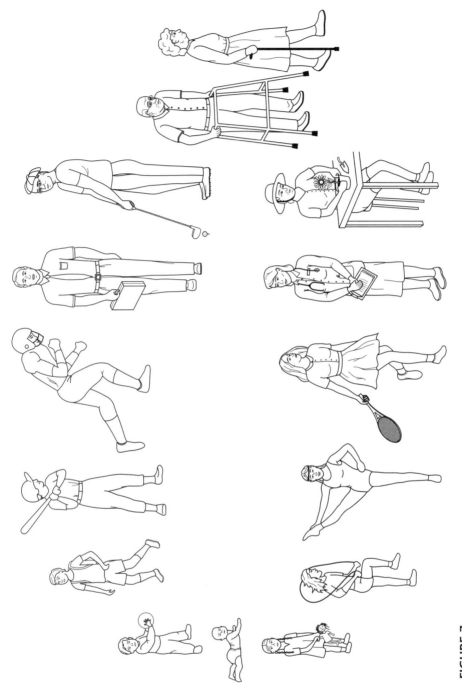

FIGURE 7

Stages of the life cycle.

In this text the first two sets are clustered together as type 1 developmental self-care requisites because both focus on self-development through stages of the life cycle. The third set is considered as the second type, or type 2 developmental self-care requisites. The discussion in the following section focuses on each of these two types.

Type 1

Type 1 developmental self-care requisites are requisites associated with those needs for self-care arising from conditions/events that normally occur at various stages of the life cycle. Requisites in the type 1 category address the promotion of human development that affects each person. If applying crisis theory to human development, conditions/events associated with type 1 developmental self-care requisites are *maturational* developmental crises. Consistent with crisis theory, successful resolution of the crisis results in progression to the next developmental task or stage. Successful resolution occurs when positive self-care actions enable the individual to cope with or manage the crisis event and resume functioning at the same or higher level.

The functional level will be less than the precrisis level if the person employs unsuccessful coping actions. This first type of developmental self-care requisite articulates very strongly with the universal self-care requisites because (1) maturational crises occur at every stage of the life cycle and for every person and (2) these affect the potential of the individual's human functioning. Sociocultural-spiritual orientation, family system, and environment basic conditioning factors strongly modify self-care actions necessary for DSCRs because conditions and resources vary greatly in different families, cultures, and geographical locations.

As stated above, type 1 developmental self-care requisites bring together the first two sets of developmental self-care requisites identified by Orem (1995, p. 197): provision of conditions to promote development and engagement in self-development. A major differentiating factor between these two sets is the personal involvement of self in the self-care actions necessary to meet the self-care requisite. In the first set the involvement of self is primarily one of recipient and respondent (dependent care recipient) to the actions of others providing care. Providers of dependent care (dependent care agents) must perform, supplement, or complement, actions that will meet and promote the natural development of the dependent care receipient and, when possible, foster increasing independence and involvement in self-care. To meet these self-care requisites, actions should be directed toward the following conditions (Orem, 1995, pp. 196–197):

- Provision and maintenance of resources (e.g., air, water, and food) and conditions (physical, emotional, and environmental) essential for:

1. Maintenance and development of life processes and human structure and functioning (both cognitive, affective, and physical)
2. Development of feelings of trust, security, safety, and being cared for
- Prevention of sensory deprivation or sensory overload
- Provision for development of self-care agency, including social skills, interaction skills, and living skills
- Provision for development of a sense of self and personhood
- Prevention of fear, anxiety, and anger through control and regulation of environmental conditions

In the second set the person is capable of actively engaging self in the deliberate action for promoting development and maturation. Orem (1995, p. 198) specified conditions for promoting self-development, and these focused self-care actions on the following:

- Seeking understanding, through reflection and introspection, of and about self, others, relationships, values and attitudes
- Seeking to understand one's own emotions and feelings and those of others about life, objects, persons—thus achieving acceptance of self and gaining insights about persons, objects, and life
- Using talents and interests effectively and productively to work in and contribute to society
- Engaging in goal and value clarification in situations in which one is personally involved
- Acting responsibly in accord with one's roles and self-ideal and self-expectations
- Seeking understanding of the value of actions associated with the attainment of positive emotions such as joy, humor, inquisitiveness, love, and spirituality
- Seeking understanding of the value of actions associated with the reduction or mitigation of negative emotions such as guilt, conflict, and anger
- Promoting positive mental health including functional self-awareness as a person in a community and self as reality based in daily living

Examples
In the following examples of a particularized self-care requisite of type 1 developmental self-care requisites, the universal self-care requisites with which the particularized developmental self-care requisite statement closely articulates are indicated in the brackets. Stages of the life cycle are strongly associated with chronological age. Therefore the influence of age as a basic conditioning factor on the origin of action in the developmental self-care requisites accounts for the inclusion of age group in parentheses before the particularized self-care requisite statement.

- (Infant) **Suckles from bottle easily**
  [Food, water, normalcy]
- (Teen) **Interacts with both male and female members of peer group**
  [Solitude and social interaction, normalcy]
- (Elder) **Participates in group activities in living unit**
  [Solitude and social interaction, activity and rest, normalcy]

Type 2

Type 2 developmental self-care requisites are those requisites associated with needs arising from specific conditions and events that may adversely affect development. Such conditions/events are unique to each individual's life experience and may occur at any stage in the life cycle; sometimes they may occur more than once in the individual's life. These conditions/events do not occur necessarily in the life of every individual: some people never experience the types of crisis events that others face. If applying crisis theory to human development, conditions/events associated with type 2 developmental self-care requisites are *situational* developmental crises. Successful resolution of the crisis results in progression to a level of functioning equal to or greater than that preceding the crisis event. An adverse effect results when the individual fails to cope successfully with the crisis event. Actions individuals take in relation to type 2 developmental self-care requisites may be directed toward promoting behaviors or providing conditions intent on (1) minimizing, mitigating, or overcoming any adverse effects of the condition or event or (2) preventing the occurrence of adverse effects.

EXERCISE

Maturation and Developmental Self-Care Requisites

For each of the following age groups, identify an action demand (i.e., some action taken or behavior evidenced) associated with the developmental level of persons typically in that age group. Remember, focus the action toward the behaviors necessary for meeting developmental tasks. You may use one or more developmental theories (e.g., Erikson, Piaget):

1. Adolescent, 14-year-old _____

_____

2. Child, 5-year-old _____

_____

3. Adult, 45-year-old _____

_____

Orem (1995, p. 199) offered a partial list of the types of conditions/events that may result in type 2 developmental self-care requisites:

- Educational deprivation
- Inadequate or difficult social adaptation
- Failure in healthy individuation
- Losses of significant others (relatives or friends), possessions, or status
- Poor health, disability, possible or impending death
- Oppressive living conditions

Examples

In the following examples of particularized self-care requisites (action demand statements) of type 2 developmental self-care requisites, the condition/event precedes the action statement in parentheses, and articulations with other self-care requisites (universal or health deviation) are indicated in brackets.

- (Rape) **Participates in a rape group therapy program**
  [Normalcy, solitude and social interaction, health deviation self-care requisite 3]
- (Teen pregnancy) **Seeks home–bound tutoring for latter part of pregnancy**
  [Normalcy, solitude and social interaction]
- (Job loss) **Consults job relocation program assisting workers of the closing factory**
  [Solitude and social interaction, normalcy]

Health Deviation Self-Care Requisites

Health deviation self-care requisites (HDSCRs) associated with those human needs arising from (1) genetic and constitutional defects, (2) human structural and functional defects or disabilities, or (3) effects of medical diagnostic and treatment measures (Orem, 1995, pp. 200-202). Health deviation self-care requisites are those needs related to (1) illness, injury, defect, or disability that may be either physical or mental in origin or result or (2) the medical treatment prescribed. These requisites represent new or different action demands that may be of temporary or long-term duration; health deviation self-care requisites are not normally present in the absence of illness, injury, disability, or disease. Clearly, the basic conditioning factors of health state and health care system are very important modifiers in health deviation self-care requisites (Orem, 1995, p. 202).

In the presence of alterations in health state, new or different needs and care measures are evident; these new requisites are health deviation self-care requisites. Individuals must first acknowledge that "something" is wrong, although they may or may not know or understand what is

E X E R C I S E

Situational Impact on Developmental Self-Care Requisites

PART I

For each of the following conditions or events, identify an action demand (i.e., some action taken or behavior evidenced) that can aid in preventing or minimizing the deleterious effects of the condition/event in a person of your age and developmental level:

1. Homeless _____

_____

2. Laid off work _____

_____

3. Mugged _____

_____

PART II

The following situation attempts to illustrate concepts about type 2 developmental self-care requisites. In the life cycle of many individuals, persons experience the death of a parent. The nature, impact, and demands of such a crisis event are different for individuals when it occurs at different points in the life cycle. (NOTE: Some individuals will never experience such an event as they themselves may die before their parents.)

Discuss the impact of such an event on the following individuals:

1. 8-year-old _____

_____

2. 25-year-old _____

_____

3. 59-year-old _____

_____

What are some self-care actions for meeting care demands associated with the same situation for the same individuals?

1. 8-year-old _____

_____

2. 25-year-old _____

_____

3. 59-year-old _____

_____

wrong. Acknowledgment of something being wrong motivates persons to seek ways in which to remedy the problem or, at least, those symptoms associated with it. Initially, persons look to their own knowledge and action repertoires when attempting to deal with problems, especially those problems with slower onset and milder changes. Persons must seek assistance from external sources when they can no longer address the problem themselves. In this way, they can learn or acquire necessary care actions from another.

Health deviation self-care requisites also articulate with the universal and developmental self-care requisites. States of health deviation often affect life processes or level of functioning. The quantity or quality of a care measure may alter, or the care measure itself may alter or change, to meet the changed status. Particularization of health deviation self-care requisites addresses actions intended to meet one (or more) of the six identified health deviation self-care requisites. Often a particularized health deviation self-care requisite statement also "overlaps" with one or more of the universal or developmental self-care requisites and other health deviation self-care requisites. The following two examples may illustrate this point:

1. Each day a person takes a warfarin (Coumadin) dose. This person is acting to follow a prescribed treatment plan (HDSCR 3) and preventing hazards (USCR 7).
2. Because of symptoms of a "common cold" and the antihistamine the person is taking, this person increases daily fluid intake by 500 to 1000 ml. This person is acting to follow a prescribed treatment plan (HDSCR 3), to mitigate a side effect of that treatment plan (HDSCR 4), and to alter fluid intake (USCR 2).

The six types of health deviation self-care requisites identified by Orem (1995, pp. 201-202) are:

1. Seeking and securing appropriate medical assistance (1) in the event of known, suspected, or anticipated exposure to known or suspected pathogens or (2) in the presence or anticipated presence of pathological conditions or defects (physical or mental)
2. Being aware of and attending to the effects and results of the health deviation (i.e., the effects and manifestations of the illness, injury, defect, disability, or the failure to prevent these)
3. Carrying out the prescribed measures necessary to diagnose, treat, prevent, or rehabilitate
4. Being aware of, attending to, or regulating the uncomfortable or adverse effects of the prescribed diagnostic, therapeutic, preventive, rehabilitative measures

5. Modifying self-concept to accept one's changed or altered health state and the necessary forms of health care
6. Learning to live with effects of the health deviation and the effects of the treatment measures

Examples

Each of the six health deviation self-care requisites is presented below with an example of a particularized self-care requisite focusing on that requisite. Action verbs in each particularized self-care requisite statement denote the general method (i.e., the usual way or expected way) of acting to achieve the purposes of self-care (i.e., self-care requisites).

- **HDSCR 1:** Go to emergency department when chest pain persists and shortness of breath develops.
- **HDSCR 2:** Record time and pattern of temperature elevations during "flu" episode.
- **HDSCR 3:** Take 650 mg of Tylenol when temperature exceeds 38.5° C.

EXERCISE

Relationships of Universal and Health Deviation Self-Care Requisites

In the event of illness or injury, new requisites for self-care are added to daily needs for self-care. As a result, self-care actions normally taken to meet universal or common requisites may change or alter. Assume that you have just come down with a moderately severe respiratory infection, a "bad common cold." Given that assumption, list at least one "new" need for self-care and self-care action that results from this kind of change in your health state for each of the universal self-care requisite categories.

1. Air _____
2. Water _____
3. Food _____
4. Elimination _____
5. Activity and rest _____
6. Solitude and social interaction _____
7. Prevention of hazards _____
8. Normalcy _____

- **HDSCR 4:** Record occurrences of insulin shock for 1 week follow-ing change in insulin dosage (for a patient with diabetes).
- **HDSCR 5:** Talk openly with other cancer patients about feelings about loss of hair from chemotherapy.
- **HDSCR 6:** Participate in Wheelchair Olympics.

Articulations Among Self-Care Requisites

Interrelationships among the self-care requisites are evident. The previous discussion described the close relationships among the universal and the developmental self-care requisites. It emphasized relationships among the universal, developmental, and health deviation self-care requisites. Most

EXERCISE

Articulation of Self-Care Requisites

For each of the six health deviation self-care requisites, an example of a particularized health deviation self-care requisite is given. For each exam-ple, identify articulations or relationships with and among other universal and developmental self-care requisites. Write the related universal and de-velopmental self-care requisites you have identified on the line below each example enclosed in brackets and preceded by ✎⊐. (NOTE: The first one has been completed as an example and is preceded by ☞.)

1. **HDSCR 1:** Go to emergency room when chest pain persists and short-ness of breath develops.

    ☞   [Air, activity and rest, prevention of hazards, normalcy]

2. **HDSCR 2:** Record time and pattern of temperature elevations during flu episode.

    ✎⊐ [_____]

    _____

3. **HDSCR 3:** Take 650 mg of Tylenol when temperature exceeds 38.5° C.

    ✎⊐ [_____]

    _____

4. **HDSCR 4:** Record occurrences of insulin shock for 1 week following change in insulin dosage (for patient with diabetes).

    ✎⊐ [_____]

    _____

continued

5. **HDSCR 5:** Talk openly with other cancer patients about feelings about loss of hair from chemotherapy.

✍ [_____]

_____

_____

6. **HDSCR 6:** Participate in Wheelchair Olympics.

✍ [_____]

_____

_____

EXERCISE

Articulating Self-Care Requisites

In the exercise below, there is a column for each of the three categories of self-care requisites (i.e., universal [USCRs], developmental [DSCRs], and health deviation [HDSCRs]). For each action demand statement (particularized self-care requisite [PSCR]), place the number(s) for each applicable self-care requisite. (See pp. 43-44 and 54-55 of requisites in self-care requisite categories of USCR and HDSCR. For DSCR, designate whether type 1 or 2 [see pp. 49 and 51]). While not all types of self-care requisites will be evident in every action statement, usually more than one is associated with an action demand statement.

The answer to number 1 is provided as an example.

Action Demand Statement: Particularized Self-Care Requisite (PSCR)	USCR	DSCR	HDSCR
1 (Infant) Nurse at each breast for 10 minutes at each of six to eight daily feedings	2, 3, 4, 5, 6, 8	1	(None)
2 (Adult, postoperative) Deep-breathe and cough three times every 2 hours when awake the first 24 hours after surgery			
3 (Child, leukemia) Use tell-a-story with self-drawn pictures about what it means to be in the hospital			
4 (Adult, anticoagulant) Contact doctor's office for Protime test whenever any kind of bleeding episode occurs			
5 (Adult, pregnant) Consume balanced 2500-calorie diet, high in iron and fiber, daily			

USCR = Universal self-care requisite.
DSCR = Developmental self-care requisite.
HDSCR = Health deviation self-care requisite.

health deviations (whether physical or mental) affect the "normal" patterns of physical and psychosocial functioning as addressed by the universal and developmental self-care requisites. The needs that arise as a result of health deviation (the HDSCRs), then, interrelate and interlock with both the universal and developmental self-care requisites. This is consistent with the concept of total human functional integrity.

There are also interrelationships evident within each category of self-care requisites. For example, the amount and type of fluids may also influence the caloric intake for the requisite of food or may influence urine or bowel elimination. Another example is that activity may affect the intake of a sufficient amount of air. An example illustrates interrelationships among health deviation self-care requisites: taking of insulin requires monitoring the effects of too much or too little insulin in the body (HDSCRs 2, 3, and 4).

Composing Particularized Self-Care Requisite Statements

Forming statements of the specific action demands necessary for meeting a self-care requisite help to understand what and how much needs to be done. Specifics of the action demand statement require application of knowledge

EXERCISE

Components of Particularized Self-Care Requisite Statements

Because a particularized self-care requisite denotes a statement of self-care action, all particularized self-care requisite statements begin with an action verb and the subject is always assumed to be the self-care agent. Further "particularization" of the action for the particularized self-care requisite statement occurs with the addition of qualifiers and quantifiers that modify or specify the nature or duration of the needed action. For this particularized self-care requisite statement (see Figure 8): "Eat 1500-calorie balanced diet, low in fats, in three meals and one snack until weight reduction of 20 lb achieved," identify the following:

1. Action verb:
2. Qualifiers:
   a. Time _____
   b. Amount _____
   c. Duration _____
   d. Quality _____
   e. Other _____

and application of the self-care agent's basic conditioning factors. The statement should begin with an action verb that serves to emphasize that action will occur. Knowledge of the general method for meeting the requisite in the situation facilitates selection of the most appropriate verb (see Figure 8). For example, the usual way or general method to meet the requisite for sufficient water intake is "to drink" (by glass or cup). Alternative general methods exist when this method is not possible or applicable because of the influence of basic conditioning factors. Examples might be that a newborn is "to suckle from breast" or an ill adult is "to consume by gastrostomy tube." The action demand is further "particularized" by adding qualifiers and quantifiers such as time, duration, amount, degree, and quality. Knowledge of the general method and which qualifiers are necessary to fully specify the type and amount of action arise from (1) an understanding of the conditioning/modifying influences of basic conditioning factors, especially age, developmental state, and health state, and (2) knowledge about care measures to meet self-care requisites. Knowledge about care actions comes from scientific fields (natural and social sciences), common sense, and experiential learning.

Once all elements of the action demand have been particularized, the resultant statement (i.e., action verb along with qualifiers/conditioners) is a particularized self-care requisite (Orem, 1995, pp. 11a, 111, 188, 270). A particularized self-care requisite is a specific, individualized statement of the action needed to meet the self-care requisite. Once formulated, a particularized self-care requisite indicates the specifics about the general self-care

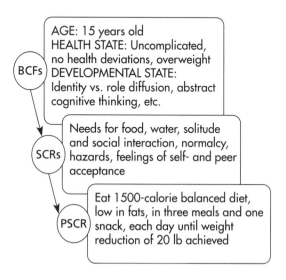

FIGURE 8

Particularized self-care requisites (PSCRs) arise from examinations of the self-care requisites (SCRs) and basic conditioning factors (BCFs).

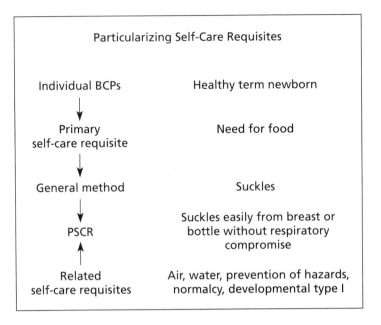

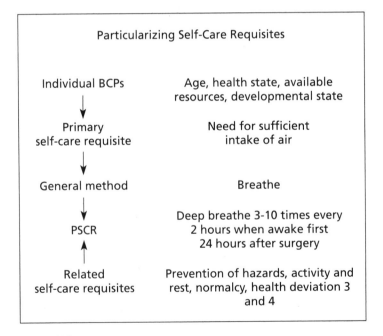

FIGURE 9

More examples of particularizing self-care requisites.

requisite while incorporating the influences of the basic conditioning factors (Figures 8 and 9).

Therapeutic Self-Care Demand

Therapeutic self-care demand (TSCD) is the *summation* (or totality) of self-care *actions* to be performed for some duration of time and in some location to meet self-care requisites particularized for a person (Orem, 1995, pp. 111-112, 186-190, 435). Achievement of therapeutic self-care means that the outcome of the selected action must be therapeutic. Therapeutic self-care demand addresses the ultimate goal of self-care: to maintain or achieve optimal health and well-being. As stated previously, particularized self-care requisites are the purposes for self-care; they represent the need for self-care and the related care actions. Therapeutic self-care demand, as an entity, is the collective set of self-care actions particularized for an individual and deemed necessary at any one point in time to achieve/accomplish therapeutic self-care. The collective set of all necessary self-care actions (represented by particularized self-care requisite statements), then, constitutes the total demand for self-care (Figure 10). When identified and stated, the totality of actions necessary for self-care (therapeutic self-care demand) constitutes a *prescription for self-care*. Individuals meet this prescription for self-care with varying degrees of effectiveness.

Consistent with the concept of self-care as deliberate action, before selecting and initiating action, one must know the needs or purposes for self-care. The performance of self-care requires that persons be able to determine the care needed. Persons engaged in self-care particularize the multiple and varied needs for self-care. They determine priorities and order requisite actions. Thus persons are actively engaged in the determination of their therapeutic self-care demand. Nurses who are actively engaged in assisting patients in achieving self-care must also understand the requisites

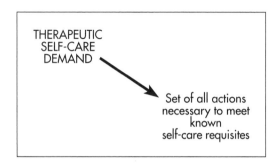

FIGURE 10
Defining therapeutic self-care demand (TSCD).

for care. They must calculate therapeutic self-care demands of persons seeking nursing assistance.

Calculation of Therapeutic Self-Care Demand

Calculation of therapeutic self-care demand is the determination of all those care actions necessary for meeting self-care requisites at a point in time. Identification of required actions alone is not enough. Ordering and prioritizing all actions and sets of actions in sequences is an essential part of determining therapeutic self-care demand. Expression of the calculated therapeutic self-care demand is in the collective statements of action required to meet all known self-care requisites at a particular point in or duration of time. As stated earlier, a statement which identifies the action or set of actions to meet a requisite is known as particularized self-care requisite. Therefore collective statements of particularized self-care requisites are appropriate representations of the calculated therapeutic self-care demand. Particularized self-care requisites are the component parts of therapeutic self-care demand (Orem, 1995, p. 205). Either emerging or existing particularized self-care requisites may focus on aspects of preventive care (Orem, 1995, p. 208).

Therapeutic self-care demand is "calculated" by particularizing the actions or set of actions necessary to meet all the universal, developmental, and health deviation of self-care requisites. Particularization of the self-care requisites (previously discussed) begins with (1) identification of the

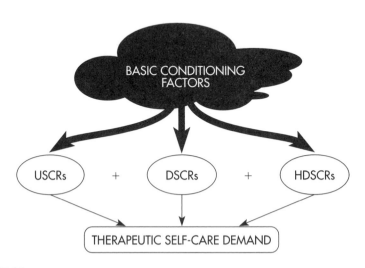

FIGURE 11

Universal, developmental, and health deviation self-care requisites (USCRs, DSCRs, and HDSCRs, respectively), as modified by basic conditioning factors, collectively equal therapeutic self-care demand (TSCD).

person's basic conditioning factors and (2) analysis of the general method and technologies of care measures associated with the requisite in light of known basic conditioning factors. From this analysis, modifiers or qualifiers of the action (i.e., time, duration, amount or degree) help specify the necessary self-care actions. Examination of all self-care requisites and identification of all self-care actions necessary to meet each of them leads to a set of particularized self-care requisites. The sum total of these particularized self-care requisites constitutes therapeutic self-care demand (see Figures 11 and 12).

Since it would be extremely arduous and lengthy to list all needed self-care actions, both nurses and clients set priorities in determining therapeutic self-care demand. For persons calculating their own therapeutic self-care demand, the process largely depends on their knowledge about self-care as developed to that point. Both knowledge and valuation of care actions and their associated outcomes affect prioritization of self-care requisites. Many self-care actions become so fixed in a regular routine of repetitious performance that they cease to exist on the conscious level as deliberate self-care (especially the intentional phase of deliberate action). Routinized self-care actions constitute habits for self-care (Orem, 1995, p. 214). These habits for self-care may come into focus at the conscious level only when there are threats or disruptions to the daily routine.

$$
\begin{aligned}
&SCR_1: \quad PSCR_{1\text{-}1}, PSCR_{1\text{-}2} \ldots PSCR_{1\text{-}y} \\
&\qquad\qquad + \\
&SCR_2: \quad PSCR_{2\text{-}1}, PSCR_{2\text{-}2} \ldots PSCR_{2\text{-}y} \\
&\qquad\qquad + \\
&SCR_3: \quad PSCR_{3\text{-}1}, PSCR_{3\text{-}2} \ldots PSCR_{3\text{-}y} \quad\Big\} \ \sum = \text{THERAPEUTIC SELF-CARE DEMAND} \\
&\qquad\qquad + \\
&\qquad\qquad \cdot \\
&\qquad\qquad \cdot \\
&\qquad\qquad \cdot \\
&SCR_y: \quad PSCR_{y\text{-}1}, PSCR_{y\text{-}2} \ldots PSCR_{y\text{-}y}
\end{aligned}
$$

FIGURE 12

Mathematical representation of calculation of therapeutic self-care demand (TSCD):
The sum of all particularized self-care requisites (PSCRs) = TSCD

Subscripts to self-care requisites (SCRs) indicate that some or all the developmental or health deviation SCRs may be included with all the universal SCRs; subscripts to PSCRs demonstrate one or more PSCRs may be necessary to address each SCR.

When nurses are involved in calculating therapeutic self-care demand, nursing knowledge, judgment, intuition, and experience facilitate the identification and prioritization of self-care requisites for patients. In nursing care situations, confirmation of calculated therapeutic self-care demand occurs via collaboration between the nurse and the client.

To summarize, therapeutic self-care demand is simply the sum of all needs for self-care and actions represented by statements of the collective set of particularized self-care requisites. The key element in calculating therapeutic self-care demand is examining, defining, and prioritizing the component parts: particularized self-care requisites (Figure 12). At any point in time, more than one particularized self-care requisite may be necessary to address the scope and complexity of each self-care requisite. When self-care is met therapeutically, self-care actions achieve or maintain the integrity of human functioning, promotion of human development, life, and well-being.

Self-Care Agency

Self-care agency (SCA) (Orem, 1995, pp. 10, 212-216, 234, 436) is the set of complex, learned, and acquired abilities (i.e., capabilities) that an individual employs when engaging in or performing self-care actions. Because of similarities in the terms, a clear understanding of the differences among the terms of self-care, self-care action, self-care agent, and self-care agency is important. Self-care is action performed in caring for self. Self-care action is a type of endeavor or activity that results in self-care. Self-care agent is the person who performs self-care. Self-care agency is the set abilities for performing the activities of self-care.

Action and the abilities for action are different. Action is the performance of an activity to accomplish something. While abilities to act are manifested in action, they are not the actions themselves. Abilities exist as potential action. They are qualities ascribed to a person's knowledge and skill repertoires. For example, a person retains the ability to read when not reading. A person retains the ability to ride a bicycle even when sitting in a classroom. The exercise of abilities or skills results in action. One cannot directly observe abilities. Looking at a person, one cannot tell if that person can read or ride a bicycle. Only if one sees that person riding a bicycle can one validate the ability to ride. "Testing" a person following a reading session is one way to validate the person's ability to read. The same ability can have differing levels of quality. For example, there is a wide range of abilities to read, from beginner to expert. This statement also applies to riding a bicycle or any other action. After observations of actions or various methods of "testing," one can make inferences about both the presence (or absence) of an ability and about the quality of the ability. Only when the potential of ability is realized as action can one make judgments about the quality of the ability. Judging quality of the ability "to read" might involve something as simple as having a person read a street sign or involve something more complex like testing reading comprehension on a college admission's test. Abilities are also specific to the action. For example, the abilities involved in reading are not the same abilities involved in riding a bicycle.

Based on the above discussion, certain properties of self-care agency (Orem, 1995, pp. 214-215) indicate the following:

- Abilities for self-care relate to self-care action.
- A person's level of performance of self-care actions is related to the quality of the persons' abilities.
- Abilities develop over time and vary in degree of adequacy from one time to another, especially under the effects of basic conditioning factors such as age and developmental state.
- Abilities develop through the various learning processes and are especially reinforced by doing/performing.
- Abilities develop within the individual's sociocultural context.

Form and Content of Self-Care Agency

Orem (1995, pp. 213-214) further described self-care agency as having both form and content. The *form* of self-care agency rests in the abilities essential for the deliberate action of self-care (Orem, 1991, p. 146). Deliberate action is the conscious, goal-oriented activity carried out in three operations: estimative, transitional, and productive (see Chapter 3). Self-care is deliberate action directed toward one's own functioning and well-being. For the deliberate action of self-care, the estimative, transitional, and productive operations of deliberate action are self-care operations (Orem, 1995, p. 221). Estimative self-care operations seek to identify (1) what self-care requisites must/should be met and why and (2) alternate ways of acting to meet those requisites. Transitional self-care operations seek to weigh and judge the alternatives resulting in a choice about what needs will be met using what actions. Actions produced by productive self-care operations address implementation of the chosen self-care actions and formulation of judgments about achievement of intended results. Abilities associated with the estimative operations are estimative abilities, those associated with transitional operations are transitional abilities, and those associated with the productive operations are productive abilities. This is just one classification system for abilities. One approach to the assessment of an individual's capacity for engaging in self-care (i.e., self-care agency) is to assess the abilities associated with the estimative, transitional, and productive self-care operations necessary for meeting the self-care requisites, as particularized for the individual. Observations of patient behavior or other assessment techniques are ways in which one can determine the abilities of the patient to identify, select, and meet a desired, expected outcome.

Qualities of abilities for the intentional phase of deliberate action (the estimative and transitional operations) do not have to be the same as the qualities of abilities of the productive phase of deliberate action (Orem, 1995, p. 234). For example, a person may be able to carry out all actions of the productive phase but lack abilities to discern and choose between two courses of action (transitional); or a person may not be able to carry out any physical actions (productive), but has active abilities related to investigation and decision-making (intentional).

Although some abilities directly related to the actions of the estimative, transitional, and productive operations related to a self-care requisite, certain common foundational abilities in individuals exist. These abilities pertain to all requisites and all persons. These abilities serve as a basis or foundation for the development or exercise of other more specialized abilities. Such foundational human abilities (Orem, 1995, p. 217) provide a supportive foundation for the estimative, transitional, and productive abilities specific to meeting a particular requisite. **Human capabilities and dispositions** (Orem, 1995, p. 217; Orem, 1979; Backscheider, 1974) is the term applied to these foundational human abilities, which include (but may not be limited to) abilities related to the following:

- Sensation and perception
- Learning and acquisition of new information
- Operational knowing and thinking
- Reflecting, reasoning, and attending to input
- Comprehending meaning
- Communication
- Decision-making
- Psychomotor skills of deliberate position and movement
- Abstraction of future events (i.e., to foresee consequences of acts)
- Understanding of self and need for self-care
- Valuing and willingness for self-care

Alteration in foundational human abilities can result in absence of estimative, transitional, or productive abilities or in drastic alterations in the development or exercise of those higher level abilities. Assessment of these foundational abilities and dispositions provides essential perspectives about the extent to which all three operations for deliberate action (estimative, transitional, and productive) can exist.

Orem (1995, p. 221) described power components that are essential for having abilities associated with the estimative, transitional, and productive self-care operations. These **power components** are human powers that are "enabling for the performance of the self-care operations" (Orem, 1995, p. 215).

These powers are necessary for and enable the development and exercise of abilities associated with the self-care operations. The 10 power components as originally described by the Nursing Development Conference Group (Orem, 1979, pp. 194-199) as stated by Orem (1995, p. 221) are listed below:

1. Ability to maintain attention and exercise requisite vigilance with respect to self as self-care agent and internal and external conditions and factors significant for self-care
2. Controlled use of available physical energy that is sufficient for the initiation and continuation of self-care operations
3. Ability to control the position of the body and its parts in the execution of the movements required for the initiation and completion of self-care operations
4. Ability to reason within a self-care frame of reference
5. Motivation (i.e., goal orientations for self-care that are in accord with its characteristics and its meaning for life, health, and well-being)
6. Ability to make decisions about care of self and to operationalize these decisions
7. Ability to acquire technical knowledge about self-care from authoritative sources, to retain it, and to operationalize it
8. A repertoire of cognitive, perceptual, manipulative, communication, and interpersonal skills adapted to the performance of self-care operations
9. Ability to order discrete self-care actions or action systems into relationships with prior and subsequent actions toward the final achievement of regulatory goals of self-care
10. Ability to consistently perform self-care operations, integrating them with relevant aspects of personal, family, and community living

The *content* of self-care agency "derives from its proper object, meeting self-care requisites, whatever those requisites are at specific moments" (Orem, 1995, p. 214). This demonstrates the direct link between the abilities of self-care agency (form) and the purposes for self-care agency (content). Abilities related to care actions are necessary to meet the therapeutic self-care demand. Exercise of abilities specific to the particularized self-care requisites produces action systems that will meet self-care requisites. The kind and amount of action necessary to meet the need identified by the self-care requisite defines the amount and types of abilities necessary to carry out that self-care action.

Understanding the form and content of self-care agency serves to organize approaches to assessment of self-care agency as the nurse or patient examines the knowledge and skill repertoires persons have and use when engaging in self-care actions intended to meet therapeutic self-care demand. Abilities associated with knowledge repertoires and skill repertoires provide one way in which to examine self-care agency (Orem, 1991, p. 147). *Knowledge repertoires* (1) pertain to the cognitive or intellectual abilities of self-care agency used to inquire, learn, retain, reason, and make decisions and (2) contribute to the valuing, prioritizing,

EXERCISE

Self-Care Agency

PART I

From the time of the appearance of the first tooth, each person has a need for dental care. Assuming an individual of your own age, health, and developmental state, identify first the abilities for self-care actions associated with each of the self-care operations for the particularized self-care requisite presented below that address an aspect of dental care.

Particularized Self-Care Requisite (PSCR)	Abilities for Self-Care Operations
Brush teeth four times daily using soft brush and fluoride toothpaste.	ESTIMATIVE
	TRANSITIONAL
	PRODUCTIVE

PART II

Development and learning of self-care occurs in the course of day-to-day living within the life context of the individual. Self-care agency, at any point in time, is modified by the individual's basic conditioning factors. For each of the basic conditioning factors, identify at least one example in which that basic conditioning factor would modify an ability in self-care agency pertaining to the particularized self-care requisite stated in Part I.

1. Age _____

2. Gender _____

3. Developmental state _____

4. Health state _____

5. Health care system _____

6. Sociocultural-spiritual orientation/family system _____

7. Patterns of living _____

8. Environment _____

9. Available resources _____

TABLE 3 Conditions and Factors Associated With Three Types of Self-Care Limitations Within Self-Care Agency

Self-Care Limitations	Sets of Conditions and Factors
Limitations of knowing	**SET 1** Changed modes of functioning that are new and are not understood; lack of fit between what one has experienced and what one is experiencing New unrecognized requirements for self-care associated with changed functional states Lack of knowledge essential for performing the operations needed to meet specific self-care requisites using specified methods and measures of care **SET 2** Impairments of sensory functioning, of perception, and of memory or attention deficits that interfere with the acquisition or recall of empirical knowledge Disturbances of human integrated functioning that adversely affect empirical consciousness, cognitive functioning, and rationality associate, for example, with (1) organic conditions that are productive of toxic states, (2) mental and emotional illness, (3) brain disorders, and (4) effects of material substances such as prescribed or unprescribed drugs **SET 3** Dispositions and orientations that result in perceptions, meanings, and appraisals of situations that are not in accord with reality Movement away from taking action to acquire new and essential learning Modes of cognitive functioning that affect mental operations associated with knowing when action is to be taken, adjusting action to existing or emerging conditions, and knowing when to stop action and modes of cognitive functioning that affect mental operations associated with organizing sets of actions into meaningful sets of sequences toward result achievement
Limitations of judging and decision-making	**SET 1** Lack of familiarity with a situation and lack of knowledge about appropriate questions for investigation Insufficient knowledge or lack of necessary skills for seeking and acquiring appropriate technical knowledge from individuals or reference materials Lack of sufficient and valid antecedent and empirical knowledge to reflect and reason within a self-care frame of reference **SET 2** Interferences with the direction and maintenance of voluntary attentions necessary to investigate situations from the perspective of self-care, for example, limitations of consciousness,

Modified with permission from Orem, D. (1995). *Nursing: Concepts of practice* (5th ed., pp. 236-239). St. Louis, MO: Mosby.

continued

Self-Care Limitations	Sets of Conditions and Factors
	SET 2—cont'd
	intense emotional states, sudden or strong likes and dislikes, overriding interests and concerns
	Inability or limited ability to imagine alternate courses of action that could be taken and the consequence of each
	SET 3
	Reluctance or refusal of individuals to investigate situations of self-care as a basis for determining what can or should be done
	Reluctance to stop reflection and make a decision once a desirable and suitable course of action is identified and understood
	Refusal to make a decision about a possible course of self-care actions or about the exercise or development of self-care agency
Limitations of engaging in result-achieving actions	**SET 1**
	Lack of knowledge or developed skills needed to operationalize decisions about self-care
	Lack of resources for self-care
	SET 2
	Lack of sufficient energy for sustained action in the intentional and productive phases of self-care as deliberate action
	Inability or limited ability to control body movements in the performance of required actions in either or both phases of self-care
	Inability or limited ability of individuals to attend to themselves as self-care agents and to exercise vigilance with respect to existing and changing internal and external conditions
	SET 3
	Lack of interest in meeting self-care requisites
	Lack of desire to meet perceived needs for self-care
	Inadequate goal orientation and values placed on self-care that do not sustain engagement in the investigative and productive phases of self-care essential for knowing and meeting therapeutic self-care demands
	SET 4
	Family members' or others' deliberate interferences with the performance of the courses of action necessary for individuals to know and meet their therapeutic self-care demands
	Patterns of personal or family living that restrict engagement in self-care operations
	Lack of social support systems needed to sustain individuals when self-care is complex, time consuming, and stressful
	Crisis situations in the family or household that interfere with self-care
	Disaster situations that interfere with engagement in self-care and with the usual ways for meeting self-care requisites

and persevering essential for meeting requisites for self-care. *Skill reper-toires* pertain to the person's cognitive, perceptual, manipulative, communication, or interpersonal abilities. These abilities of self-care agency facilitate engagement in self-care actions and include such abilities associated with attending to details, performing physical movement and manipulation for self-care actions, and monitoring self-care actions and results of self-care actions.

Assessment of self-care agency is essential before nurses can determine why and how persons can be helped by nursing. After assessing which abilities are present, judgments about agency pertain to development, operability, and adequacy. Judgments about development of abilities include assessing whether (1) the abilities are absent (undeveloped), (2) the abilities are present, but of insufficient quality (underdeveloped), or (3) the abilities are present and of sufficient quality (developed). Judgments about operability of abilities include (1) operable, if present, and exercise of abilities is both wise and safe and (2) inoperable, if present, but conditions or factors prohibit or make the exercise of those abilities unsafe or unwise. Finally, judgments about adequacy of self-care agency address the adequacy of abilities to meet the self-care requisite. If abilities are present and operable and are sufficient to meet the self-care requisite, then self-care agency is adequate.

If abilities are judged inadequate, there are evident limitations in performing self-care. Self-care limitations represent those restrictions that prohibit the performance of self-care action (Orem, 1995, p. 236). Self-care limitations are directly related to deficiencies of self-care agency and lead to self-care deficits. Three categories of self-care limitations are identified: limitations of knowing, limitations of judging and decision-making, and limitations of engaging in result–achieving actions (Orem, 1995, pp. 236-240). Table 3 presents conditions and factors associated with these three types of self-care limitations.

Self-Care Deficit

The theory of self-care deficit (Orem, 1995, pp. 174-175), which is the second constituent theory of the self-care deficit theory of nursing (SCDTN), identifies the types of relationships that can exist between the two patient variables of therapeutic self-care demand (TSCD) and self-care agency (SCA) (Orem, 1995, p. 178). The emphasis on what ways self-care requisites (demand) and abilities to perform care to meet self-care requisites (agency) relate is an important aspect of this theory. Three possible relationships (Orem, 1995, p. 240) between these two entities exist:

1. Demand is equal to abilities (TSCD = SCA)
2. Demand is less than abilities (TSCD < SCA)
3. Demand is greater than abilities (TSCD > SCA)

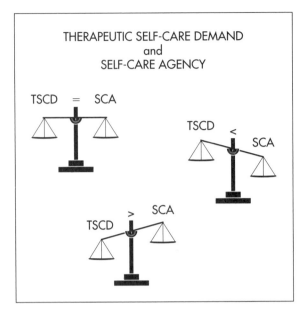

FIGURE 13
Relationships between therapeutic self-care demand (TSCD) and self-care agency (SCA).

In the first two, the relationships show self-care (agency) abilities are at least adequate or more than adequate to meet the self-care requisites. The balance between the two entities is equal where each has equal weight or the balance is one in which abilities exceed or outweigh demand (Figure 13). In both situations persons are able to and do meet self-care requisites through the exercise of their own existing abilities. There is no *deficit relationship* between the two entities. Persons whose self-care abilities (agency) meet or exceed their self-care requisites can adequately and successfully accomplish self-care and, as such, are of no legitimate concern to nurses.

Self-care deficit (Orem, 1995, pp. 10, 175, 240–242) pertains to the third type of relationship between the therapeutic self-care demand and self-care agency. This last relationship depicts one in which all or some of the self-care requisites are not met because of insufficient self-care abilities for carrying out care measures or lack of operability of existing self-care abilities. The result is failure to accomplish therapeutic self-care. By definition, then, **self-care deficit (SCD)** exists when the therapeutic self-care demand (TSCD) exceeds the abilities of self-care agency (SCA): SCD = TSCD > SCA. Self-care deficits can be either existing or projected. An **existing self-care deficit** is one in which the self-care abilities (agency) for self-care requisites are currently inadequate to meet the current self-care requisites (demand). An example of an existing self-care deficit is an individual having difficulty managing postoperative pain in the first hours following surgery. A **projected self-care deficit** is one in which the current self-care abilities (agency) for self-care requisites are, at that point in time, inadequate for an anticipated or known future change in the therapeutic self-care demand. An example of a projected self-care deficit is an individual, scheduled for surgery, who has no knowledge of the postoperative care needs or practices; teaching about the postoperative care before surgery ensures improved recovery following surgery.

Nurses' diagnostic efforts lead to detection of self-care deficits. First, assessment focuses on defining and specifying the components of therapeutic self-care demand: the particularized self-care requisites. This leads to a prescription for self-care (i.e., what needs to be). Next, efforts focus on assessing self-care abilities and self-care limitations in relation to the particularized self-care requisites. Self-care abilities are the "plus" or asset side of self-care agency, whereas self-care limitations are the "negative" or debit side (Orem, 1995, p. 236). Self-care limitations identify what restricts or prohibits the patient "from providing the amount and kind of self-care" (Orem, 1995, p. 236) that is needed to meet the current or changing therapeutic self-care demand in a therapeutic, effective manner. Determination of self-care limitations can only occur after a close examination and assessment of patient's self-care abilities as associated with the self-care requisites. Assessing self-care agency involves the examination of the foundational abilities and dispositions, power components, and self-care abilities associated with the estimative, transitional, and productive self-care operations.

Self-care limitations are restrictions or deficiencies in knowing, in judging and decision-making, or in engaging in result-achieving actions. These three types of self-care limitations have a link to the abilities associated with the three self-care operations (estimative, transitional, and productive) (Table 4). Because of this link, assessments of self-care agency can focus on the three types of self-care limitations or on the three self-care operations. Following diagnostic efforts, nurses' efforts center on determining the relationship between the two entities of therapeutic self-care demand and self-care agency. A deficit relationship between the two entities is a self-care deficit. Self-care limitations are the most significant determinants of self-care deficits.

Presence of self-care limitations indicates that the self-care actions directed toward meeting self-care requisites are limited because self-care abilities are not sufficient. Lack of developed self-care abilities is one reason for insufficiency. Another reason may be that it would be unwise or impossible to exercise developed or developing abilities (i.e., lack of operability). When the person has self-care limitations, he or she is unable to carry out

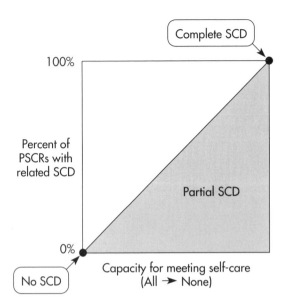

FIGURE 14
Self-care deficits (SCDs) can be partial or complete. *PSCR,* Particularized self-care requisite.

TABLE 4 Linking Types of Self-Care Limitations With Self-Care Operations	
Types of Self-Care Limitations	**Self-Care Operations**
Knowing	Estimative
	Transitional
	Productive
Judging and decision-making	Transitional
	Productive
Engaging in result-achieving actions	Estimative
	Productive

the required self-care actions necessary to meet therapeutic self-care demand. Failure to meet some or all of the requisites of therapeutic self-care means that therapeutic self-care is not met.

Self-care deficits could arise from any of the multiple particularized self-care requisites making up therapeutic self-care demand. Therefore, at one time, a person could have one or more deficits. When 100% of all particularized

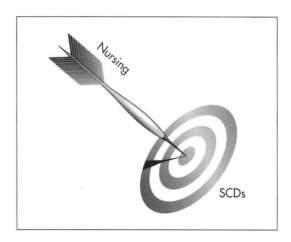

FIGURE 15

Self-care deficits (SCDs) are the targets for nursing care.

self-care requisites evidence a deficit relationship, self-care deficits are *complete* (Figure 14). In such a case, the individual evidences no capacity for engaging in the deliberate action of self-care, for example, a comatose patient. For anything less than 100%, self-care deficits are *partial* (Orem, 1995, p. 240).

Nursing, as a socially recognized and organized health service, seeks to deliver nursing care to patients who demonstrate a need for nursing. The ultimate goal of nursing is to assure achievement of therapeutic self-care (Orem, 1995, pp. 316, 323). To this end, nursing's concern is for persons with health-derived or health-related self-care deficits. These persons, then, are the legitimate patients★ of nursing. A **legitimate patient of nursing** has existing or projected self-care deficits as evidenced by the presence of self-care limitations. Designed systems of nursing target problems posed by self-care deficits (Figure 15). Nursing care focuses on eliminating self-care deficits by (1) reducing the need, (2) eliminating action limitations through supporting the development or exercise of self-care abilities (agency), or (3) reducing the need so that it is manageable. In situations where development or mobilization of self-care agency is not possible, nursing care must focus efforts on performing care actions for clients.

★The use of the word *patient* here represents a broad, generic term for the unit of service in nursing. The patient may be either an individual or a multiperson unit (couple, family, group/aggregate, or community).

Dependent Care

The theory of self-care/dependent care (Orem, 1995, pp. 170-174) introduces the concept of dependent care as distinct from the concept of self-care. Yet, there is a clear relationship between the two concepts (see Chapter 2). The phrase "dependent care" appears often throughout the discussion of the three constituent theories of self-care deficit theory of nursing. A simple slash mark usually pairs the phrase "dependent care" with the phrase "self-care" so that they equal a single noun in a sentence. Both self-care and dependent care represent action systems produced when deliberate action is directed toward meeting requisites for self-care. **Dependent care** is the practice of actions that an individual initiates and performs continuously on behalf of another who for reasons of health state or developmental state cannot perform some or all of required self-care actions (Orem, 1995, pp. 9, 435). The intent of dependent care is to regulate and promote human functioning and human development and to contribute to the maintenance of life, health, and well-being of the person in need of care from another. Socially dependent persons are those who require dependent care. Often, the cultural and social group norms guide identification of who is acceptably socially dependent and who is responsible for those who are socially dependent. Dependency on another may exist for a short or long duration of time; the level of dependency may change over time. Persons performing dependent care are responsible adults (e.g., parent, guardian, or designated family member[s]) typically caring for children or persons with disabling physical or mental conditions.

Dependent care is a concept parallel to that of self-care. Dependent care and self-care share many of the same characteristics. The major difference between the two concepts is *who* is the target of care actions. Self-care is the production and practice of activities directed toward oneself or one's environment to regulate one's own functioning and development and maintain one's life, health, and well-being (Orem, 1995, p. 95). In self-care, the target for care actions is always self, while in dependent care, the target for care actions is another person (most often a family member) who relies on others for care on an ongoing basis. The following discussion focuses on major similarities and differences between self-care and dependent care.

- Dependent care is *like* self-care in the following ways:
    1. Dependent care is deliberate action with estimative, transitional, and productive operations.
    2. Dependent care is an action system in which discrete actions are logically ordered and sequentially performed.
    3. Dependent care is purpose-oriented action (i.e., it is action intended to meet known self-care requisites of the person receiving care). The

actions of the dependent care system can and do meet these requisites for care.

4. Dependent care is action performed by persons having specialized abilities (i.e., dependent care agency).
5. Dependent care actions and needs are conditioned and modified by the basic conditioning factors.
6. Dependent care is learned in a sociocultural context; this emphasizes that dependent care is not instinctual nor is it haphazard. Education for dependent care takes place most often in the family-social setting.
7. Dependent care can be either ineffective or effective. This means that the action taken for care may not produce the desired effect or intended outcome.
8. Dependent care can be either therapeutic or nontherapeutic. This means that the end product of the intended action may or may not be positive.
9. Dependent care is necessary to meet requisites for care in those acknowledged by society as legitimately dependent.
10. Dependent care has new or altered needs because of the presence of health deviations.

- Dependent care is *unlike* self-care in the following ways:
  1. Dependent care is *not* performed for one's self; actions are performed for the benefit of another. As such, it requires interaction between at least two persons.
  2. Dependent care is *not* intended to meet one's own self-care requisites; the intent is to meet the self-care requisites of another.
  3. Although dependent care is continuous over time, it is ideally intended to give way to self-care (especially for children). Some dependent care systems are lifelong or, at least, what constitutes the remainder of a person's life; others may have specified duration, for example, when the person's body cast is removed. The emphasis of this point is that self-care is the ideal goal and each dependent care system should be evaluated regarding its necessity and longevity: at what point, if any, will dependent care no longer be needed?

Because self-care and dependent care are different but parallel concepts, conceptual terminology specific to dependent care and dependent care systems helps to maintain the similarities and distinctions between the two. Exploration of these concepts and terms helps to clarify further similarities and differences between self-care and dependent care. Conceptual clarification contributes to building of a conceptual model specific to dependent care. Terminology parallels that developed for self-care. The following discussion focuses on the terms: dependent care recipient, dependent care agent, dependent care agency, and dependent care deficits.

Dependent care recipient (DCR)★ is the person in need of and receiving dependent care provided by another person(s). Children, disabled spouses, or elderly parents might be examples of persons in need of dependent care. There are three key elements about dependent care recipients. First, dependent care recipients are persons who legimately need assistance in meeting one, some, or all self-care requisites because of the presence of one or more self-care deficits. This means provision of required care on a continuing basis usually by one or more persons of a family or as designated by society is necessary. In this system of care, there are definitions of roles as to who will be the recipient and who will be the provider.

Second, the self-care requisites are those of the dependent care recipient (Orem, 1995, p. 160), not the dependent care agent. Therefore in dependent care systems the therapeutic self-care demand should always be calculated in terms of the dependent care recipient (just as in self-care). In calculating therapeutic self-care demand for a dependent care recipient, generation of particularized self-care requisite statements are action oriented and specific to the dependent care recipient. Calculation of therapeutic self-care demand addresses the ideal of what is necessary for care to be therapeutic and effective while making no judgments about whether or not someone other than the dependent care recipient should perform the action. Therapeutic self-care demand specifies the needed care actions. Judgments about who can or should perform care actions are made only when comparisons of demand and abilities determine self-care deficits.

Third, a dependent care recipient often has some capacity for self-care (i.e., only partial deficit). As such, the dependent care recipient's self-care system is operative and must be coordinated with the dependent care system to produce a harmonious system of care. In situations where self-care deficits are partial, dependent care agents and dependent care recipients must work together cooperatively. Promoting the ideal of moving toward self-care in dependent care systems emphasizes that dependent care agents should be providing only care focused toward the self-care deficits of the dependent care recipient. The only situation in which dependent care systems totally replace self-care systems is one in which self-care deficits of the dependent care recipient are complete. This third element stresses the complexity of dependent care systems: the cooperative efforts of the interaction of the persons involved and the two systems of care.

★*Dependent care recipient* is a term proposed by this author; Orem (1995, p. 200) refers to the receiver of dependent care. Creation of this term helps to differentiate the "participants" in the dependent care system: recipient versus agent.

Dependent care agent (Orem, 1995, pp. 200, 243-244) is the person performing the actions of dependent care continuously, over time. This person is typically a family member or friend (e.g., mother, grandparent, sibling, or legal guardian). Persons responsible for dependent care are also responsible for their own self-care actions. Thus they must learn to coordinate and articulate the actions for their own self-care with those actions necessary for the performance of dependent care. For example, the mother of a newborn must care for the baby 24 hours a day and yet meet her own self-care requisites for rest and sleep. The number and type of care measures that the dependent care agent must provide to meet self-care requisites of the dependent care recipient determine the "burden" of dependent care that is met by the dependent care agent.

Dependent care agency (DCA) (Orem, 1995, pp. 10, 171, 212, 242-243) is the complex set of abilities of the dependent care agent to carry out the required dependent care actions. The concept of dependent care agency is parallel to that of self-care agency.

- Dependent care agency is *like* self-care agency in several ways:
  1. Dependent care agency, like self-care agency, focuses on abilities for carrying out care actions.
  2. Dependent care agency consists of foundational capabilities and dispositions, power components, and abilities associated with estimative, transitional, and productive operations of deliberative action.
  3. Dependent care agency is modified by the basic conditioning factors.
  4. Dependent care agency is assessed by examining the abilities associated with the estimative, transitional, and productive operations of deliberate action.
  5. Dependent care agency may be a combination of abilities and limitations. Dependent care limitations are analogous to self-care limitations in that they are restrictions or limitations in the performance of action.
  6. Dependent care agency consists of abilities that are learned and developed over time within the family system and sociocultural spiritual context and, sometimes, through more formal processes of education.
- Dependent care agency is *unlike* self-care agency in several ways:
  1. The abilities of dependent care agency concentrate on the actions necessary for dependent care that may be similar to or different from those of self-care. For example, brushing your own teeth is similar yet different from brushing the teeth of another. This difference is even more notable if the other person is unconscious.
  2. Self-care agency focuses on the deliberate action of self-care and dependent care agency focuses on the deliberate action of dependent care. When exercised, dependent care agency results in dependent care.

3. Dependent care agency is exercised for the benefit of another, requiring the interaction and mutual cooperation of at least two persons.

Dependent care deficit (DCD)★ (Orem, 1995, pp. 10-12, 171, 175) addresses the relationship between the demand for self-care (i.e., the therapeutic self-care demand [TSCD] of the dependent care recipient [DCR]) and the abilities of the dependent care agent (i.e., dependent care agency [DCA]) to produce care. Like self-care deficit, a deficit relationship in dependent care systems exists when the demand for care exceeds the abilities for care. This deficit relationship can be expressed as:

$$\text{TSCD (of DCR)} > \text{SCA (of DCR)} + \text{DCA} = \text{DCD}$$

This definition of dependent care deficit depicts a parallel relationship between the concept of self-care deficit and the concept of dependent care deficit, but it is rather simplistic and does not provide full insight into the complexities of dependent care systems. One therapeutic self-care demand is of concern, that of the recipient. Dependent care systems have two active agencies (unless there is complete self-care deficit, see above). The two agencies (sets of abilities) are that of the dependent care recipient and that of the dependent care agent. The agency of the dependent care recipient is in actuality that person's self-care agency (SCA). The relationship between the dependent care recipient and the dependent care agent is one of mutual cooperation. Dependent care agents should respect and support the dependent care recipient's efforts toward self-care; at times, the role of the dependent care agent is to teach, guide, and direct the dependent care recipient in the development and exercise of his or her own self-care agency (for example, the role relationship between parent and child). Dependent care is more complex than self-care because of these added dimensions. The following may better represent the complexity of the system of dependent care:

$$\text{TSCD (of DCR)} > \text{SCA (of DCR)} = \text{SCD}$$
$$\downarrow$$
$$\text{Demand for dependent care} > \text{DCA} = \text{DCD}$$

Summary

Basic conditioning factors influence all persons and characterize the uniqueness of each individual not only by genetic, age, and developmental differences but also by variations according to environment, lifestyle, culture,

---

★The term *dependent care deficit* is most evident in Orem's most recent work (1995); the phrase was rarely used in prior editions with little or no explanation of what is clearly meant by this term.

spirituality, interpersonal relationships (families, etc.). Assessing relevant basic conditioning factors can provide descriptions of persons engaged in self-care/dependent care (i.e., self-care agents/dependent care agents).

Self-care is deliberate action produced when the action initiated is for the purpose of influencing internal or external factors that contribute to integrated functioning and development (i.e., to health and well-being). Self-care is always performed for oneself by oneself. When one acts in caring for oneself, the term for that person is *self-care agent*.

Successful conduct of self-care depends on the individual's abilities (self-care agency) for meeting known or projected demands/needs for self-care (i.e., self-care requisites). Meeting self-care requisites means that abilities are exercised (i.e., employed or activated). Categories of self-care requisites for self-care include universal, developmental, and health deviation. Each self-care requisite is a generalization about the care needed. Interrelationships exist between and among all the self-care requisites. Particularization of self-care requisites results in specification about the type, amount, and duration of action necessary to meet the self-care requisite. Particularized self-care requisites, thus, quantify and qualify the action(s) necessary to meet needs. The collective sum of these needs, when expressed as particularized self-care requisites, constitutes therapeutic self-care demand.

The relationship between self-care agency (abilities) and the therapeutic self-care demand (requisites), both of which are conditioned/modified by basic conditioning factors, determines the quality of self-care produced. This relationship between therapeutic self-care demand (TSCD) and self-care agency (SCA) can be expressed either as a deficit relationship or not.

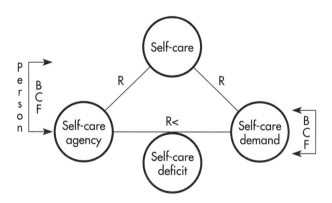

FIGURE 16

Conceptual model for concepts pertaining to self-care. *BCF* = basic conditioning factor; *R* = relationship; < = deficit relationship.

(Modified with permission from Orem D. [1995]. *Nursing: Concepts of practice* [5th ed., p. 213]. St. Louis, MO: Mosby.)

In the deficit relationship the therapeutic self-care demand (TSCD) is greater than the self-care agency (SCA) possessed or exercised by the individual (i.e., SCA < TSCD). When such a deficit relationship exists, the person is unable to carry out all the actions necessary for the accomplishment of all therapeutic self-care. In this case self-care limitations are evident and contribute to the existence of self-care deficits. Two other relationships between the therapeutic self-care demand and the self-care agency exist in which there are no deficits. Statements that represent these relationships are SCA = TSCD *or* SCA > TSCD. In both of these cases persons are able to perform and achieve therapeutic self-care without help. The conceptual model for the related concepts of self-care is presented in Figure 16.

When persons are unable to care for themselves by virtue of health state, developmental state, or age, their self-care requisites may be met (in part or whole) by assistance from guardians, parents, or family members. Such persons who are unable to meet all, most, or some of their self-care requisites are in need of and should receive dependent care that supplements and complements self-care. Persons who provide dependent care are dependent care agents and the persons they care for are dependent care recipients. Abilities of dependent care agents to provide dependent care constitute dependent care agency. In dependent care systems the focus is on meeting self-care requisites (in total known as therapeutic self-care demand) of the dependent care recipient. In dependent care systems the existence of dependent care deficits (i.e., there is a deficit relationship between agency and demand) validates a need for nursing. The conceptual model presented in Figure 17 demonstrates the complexity of conceptual relationships associated with dependent care.

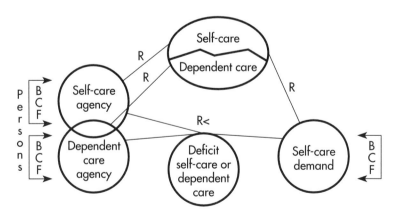

FIGURE 17

Conceptual model for concepts pertaining to dependent care. *BCF* = basic conditioning factor; *R* = relationship; < = deficit relationship.

(Modified with permission from Orem D. [1995]. *Nursing: Concept of practice* [5th ed., p. 213]. St. Louis, MO: Mosby.)

CHAPTER 5

Nursing and Nursing Systems

OUTLINE

Nursing Agency

Nursing System

Methods of Helping

Nursing Situation

   Group 1: Health Promotion Throughout the Life Cycle

   Group 2: Recovery

   Group 3: Illness of Undetermined Origin

   Group 4: Genetic and Developmental Defects and Biological Immaturity

   Group 5: Cure or Regulation

   Group 6: Stabilization of Integrated Functioning

   Group 7: Terminal Illness

KEY TERMS

Methods of helping

Nursing agency

Nurse agent

Nursing situation

Nursing system

The theory of nursing system (see Chapter 2) introduces the major nursing variable, nursing agency, and the concept of nursing system and establishes the nature of nursing as a helping service in practice situations (Orem, 1995, pp. 175-177). This embraces all the concepts introduced in the first two theories including self-care/dependent care, therapeutic self-care demand, and self-care agency/dependent care agency and self-care deficit/dependent care deficit. Nursing agency is the power of nurses for exercising developed or developing abilities for the provision of the deliberate action of nursing (Orem, 1995, p. 246). In exercising the abilities of nursing agency, nurses produce systems of care (i.e., nursing systems) designed to assist patients with health-derived or health-related self-care (dependent care) deficits. These systems of care are nursing systems. The quality of the helping service provided is also in part dependent on the willingness of the nurse to exercise nursing agency and to produce nursing in nursing situations (Orem, 1995, p. 89).

Nursing Agency

Nursing agency is the nurse variable of Orem's self-care deficit theory of nursing (SCDTN; Orem, 1995, p. 178). Nursing agency is the complex set of learned, acquired *abilities* for the deliberate action of nursing (Orem, 1995, pp. 11, 246-291, 329). Education in the specialized discipline of nursing (as provided by nursing education programs) initially develops abilities for nursing. Experience and continuing education foster the continuing development of agency over time. The complex set of abilities that make up nursing agency includes all those necessary for the design and production of nursing. Abilities operationalized aim at meeting the patient's requirements for nursing, which are associated with or arising from a wide range and variety of existing or projected self-care or dependent care deficits. Basic conditioning factors are characterizing features of persons who are nurses (Orem, 1995, p. 329). The conditioning effects of these factors influence the kinds and types of abilities possessed by a nurse, emphasizing the uniqueness of every nurse. Exercise of the abilities making up nursing agency by persons legitimately occupying the role of nurse results in the performance of nursing actions and the production of nursing care. When abilities are exercised, nurses (1) determine the need for nursing care, which is based on the presence of health-related self-care deficits or dependent-care deficits; (2) design a nursing system that subsumes a plan for the delivery of nursing care; (3) carry out that plan; and (4) judge the results of actions implemented as part of the plan of care. Nurses must possess these abilities to produce effective nursing (Orem, 1995, p. 246).

In the preceding chapter, *self-care agency* is the term used for abilities for the deliberate action of self-care. Nursing agency represents abilities for the deliberate action of nursing care. Self-care agency and nursing agency are analogous concepts. Identification of other similarities and differences between nursing agency and self-care agency is important to fully understand the two as separate concepts. Following are some major similarities and differences between nursing agency and self-care agency:

- Nursing agency is *like* or similar to self-care agency in the following ways:
  1. Abilities learned and developed over time make up nursing agency.
  2. Basic conditioning factors modify or condition the abilities of nursing agency.
  3. Assessment of nursing agency involves the examination of the abilities associated with performance of the estimative, transitional, and productive operations (as described in the concept of deliberate action). Assessment also includes human capabilities and dispositions and power components.
  4. Exercise of nursing agency results in deliberate action.
  5. Nursing agency may be assessed as a combination of abilities and limitations. This means that the person who legitimately occupies the role of nurse (i.e., **nurse agent**) has a set of abilities and a set of limitations that affect the scope of the nurse agent's ability to act in any time-specific situation. Use of the word *nurse* refers to nurse agent.
- Nursing agency is *unlike* or different from self-care agency in the following ways:
  1. The operations of deliberate action of concern for nursing agency are those related to the estimative, transitional, and productive operations of nursing care, not self-care, as a form of deliberate action.
  2. Abilities of nursing agency correspond with the social, interpersonal, and professional-technological components of the process of nursing (see Chapter 6).
  3. Abilities of nursing agency are developed and exercised for the benefit and well-being of others who are legitimate patients of nurses. The process of developing abilities requires interaction between at least two persons. Abilities for the production of nursing actions are essential components of nursing agency, but additional abilities are necessary to manage the social and interpersonal components of the interaction. This makes nursing agency more analogous to dependent care agency.
  4. The abilities making up nursing agency relate to the actions necessary for the production of nursing care; these are, at times, similar to and, at times, different from those of actions for self-care.
  5. Education programs in nursing specialize in the development and teaching of the knowledge and skills that make up nursing agency. Abilities learned via academic and experiential study of nursing provide a broader scope and more depth of scientific knowledge than those of self-care.

Again, the exercise of nursing agency results in the design, plan, and production of a nursing system that includes nursing actions necessary for protecting the nurse's health and the sustaining and promoting of health and well-being *of others*. Both nursing care and dependent care are action systems producing action for the care of others. Through the exercise of nursing agency, nurses attempt to assist patients with health–derived or health-related self-care (or dependent care) deficits (Orem, 1995, p. 247). Dependent care action systems produce dependent care to meet the self-care requisites of "family" (in the broadest sense of the term *family member[s]*). Provision of dependent care is on a continuing basis. Nurses also differ from dependent care agents because of their specialized knowledge and skills associated with the deliberate action of nursing care.

The abilities that make up nursing agency are concerned with, but are not limited to, such activities as (1) assessing and making judgments about the therapeutic self-care demand and relationships among the component self-care requisites of the therapeutic self-care demand, (2) ensuring the accomplishment of therapeutic self-care, (3) assessing and making judgments about the self-care (dependent care) agency, (4) assisting patients to exercise or develop self-care agency or protect the current self-care (dependent care) agency. Decisions made by nurses determine why and how a patient can be helped by nursing. Actions of a nurse in helping patients in various situations seek to (1) reduce or alter the demand, (2) supplement the patient's self-care (dependent care) by performing care actions the patient is unable to perform, (3) promote the development of new abilities in patients, (4) assist patients in operationalizing and exercising their own abilities, and (5) protect patients from deleterious effects that may reduce their ability to act (see Figure 18). When nurses ex-

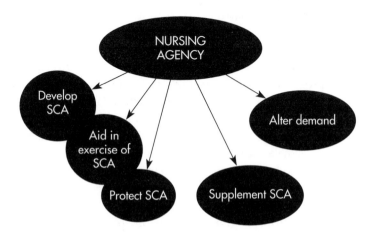

FIGURE 18

Exercised abilities of nursing agency affect both self-care agency (SCA) and therapeutic self-care demand.

ercise nursing agency to create nursing systems unique to the patient's needs and situation, the nurse is exercising creative efforts.

Nursing System

A **nursing system** is the continuing series of organized, concrete set of deliberate actions designed and performed by nurses in collaboration with the patient (either an individual or multiperson unit; Orem, 1995, pp. 302-313). Nursing systems are complex sets of nursing actions selected and produced by nurses with two goals in mind: (1) ensuring accomplishment of therapeutic self-care (i.e., achievement of therapeutic self-care demand) and (2) protecting or developing existing self-care (or dependent care) agency or assisting in the exercise of self-care (or dependent care) agency. Only nurses, through exercise of nursing agency, create and execute nursing systems. The designed nursing system represents the actions and interactions of the nurse and patient in the social, interpersonal, and technological components of the process of nursing in nursing practice (see Chapter 6). As a framework for planning, the design of the nursing system prescribes the role of the nurse and the role of the patient. Role prescription specifies what the patient will do, what the nurse will do, and what the nurse and patient will do together (Figure 19). Contracting and collaboration are important processes in the interactions between nurse and patient.

There are three types of nursing systems: supportive-educative, partly compensatory, and wholly compensatory (Orem, 1995, p. 306). The decision about what type of nursing system design is appropriate for meeting the patient's self-care (or dependent care) deficits rests on the answer to a question that addresses *who can or should perform actions necessary to meet the self-care requisites* (see Table 5 and Figure 19). Remember, nurses only address this question about legitimate patients of nursing (i.e., patients with known self-care [or dependent care] deficits).

Once selected, the nursing system serves as the basic architectural design that guides development and formulation of a plan of care. The type of nursing system selected also suggests which major methods of helping are appropriate before deciding on specific nursing actions. In this plan of care, those actions agreed on by the nurse and the patient are specifically outlined and organized. In the nursing system, accomplishment of therapeutic self-care is through the collective actions of the nurse and the patient following initiation of actions included in the plan of care. Figure 20 summarizes some of the major characteristics of nursing systems.

Methods of Helping

According to Orem (1995), "the basic design of a nursing system is a helping system" (p. 304). The main nursing actions that compose a nursing system are, in some way, helping actions. Orem (1995, p. 15) described five

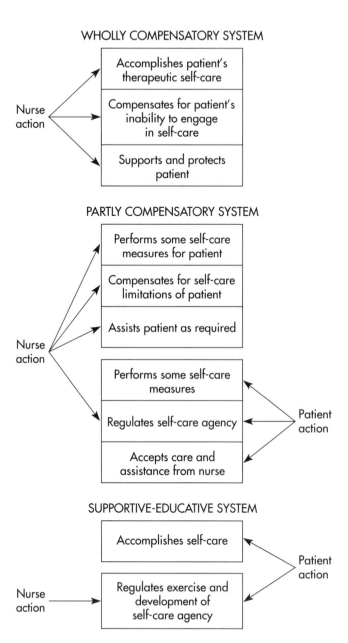

FIGURE 19

Actors in basic nursing systems. (Reprinted with permission from Orem, D. [1995]. *Nursing: Concepts of practice* [5th ed., p. 307]. St. Louis, MO: Mosby.)

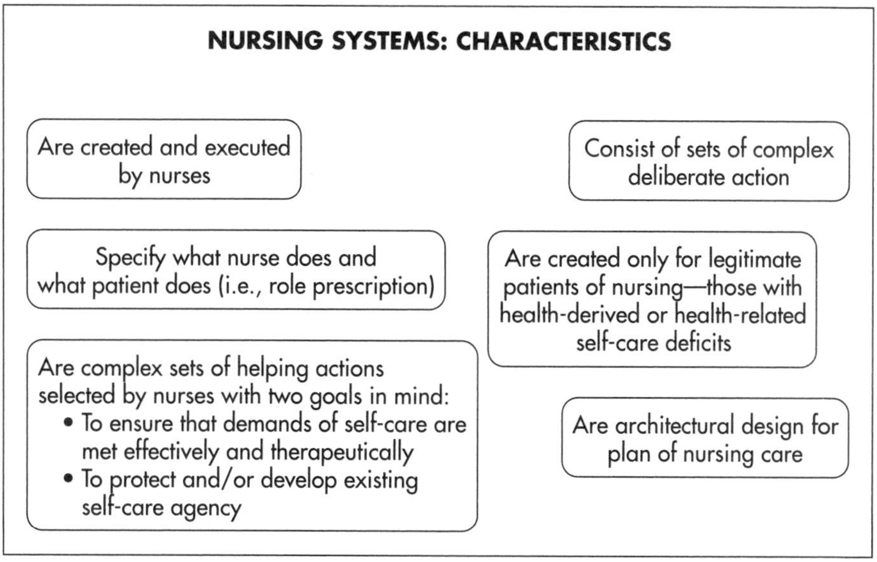

NURSING SYSTEMS: CHARACTERISTICS

Are created and executed by nurses

Consist of sets of complex deliberate action

Specify what nurse does and what patient does (i.e., role prescription)

Are created only for legitimate patients of nursing—those with health-derived or health-related self-care deficits

Are complex sets of helping actions selected by nurses with two goals in mind:
- To ensure that demands of self-care are met effectively and therapeutically
- To protect and/or develop existing self-care agency

Are architectural design for plan of nursing care

FIGURE 20
Characteristics of nursing systems.

TABLE 5 Determining What Type of Nursing System Is Appropriate		
Question	**Answer**	**Type of Nursing System**
"Who can or should perform those self-care operations [considering both phases of deliberate action] that require movement in space and controlled manipulation?" (Orem, 1995, p. 306)	Patient	Supportive-educative
	Nurse and patient	Partly compensatory
	Nurse	Wholly compensatory

general categories of helping methods; the five general methods of helping are (1) acting or doing for another, (2) guiding another, (3) supporting another, (4) providing a developmental environment, and (5) teaching another. As methods of helping, these general categories are applicable to any helping service yet are made unique to nursing through the exercise of nursing agency when applying these to patient care in nursing situations. **Methods of helping** are those general methods employed by nurses in assisting or helping patients overcome or compensate for the problems posed by self-care deficits (or dependent care deficits) (Orem, 1995, pp. 14–20). Nursing agency includes abilities to assess and determine the method of helping and related nursing actions appropriate to compensate for or overcome self-care (or dependent care) deficits. Each method of helping assists in defining the role(s) of the nurse in the nursing system and suggests more specific actions that facilitate goal achievement. In addition, methods of helping, either directly or implicitly, indicate the role of the patient (Orem, 1995, p. 286). Specific actions derived from and related to one or more of the various methods of helping come together to create a plan of care. The nursing knowledge and skills associated with methods of helping are important abilities developed as part of nursing agency through nursing education. Selection and use of methods of helping are crucial to designing nursing systems and formulating plans of care (see Chapter 6).

The following list helps to define each of the five methods of helping. Examples of actions associated with the method of helping follow each definition.

1. *Acting or doing for another.* The nurse carries out and performs those actions or care measures required for accomplishment of self-care requisites that the patient cannot perform. Patients are unable to perform these actions or it is unwise that they do. The performance of action is part of the second phase (the productive phase) of deliberate action and necessitates psychomotor skills and manipulative movement. When at all possible, the nurse should include the patient in the first phase (the intentional phase) of deliberate action: knowledge seeking efforts about self-care requisites and decision-making. Sometimes because of the nature of the illness, injury, defect, or disability, the patient cannot engage even in the first phase of deliberate action.

   EXAMPLES: Performing oral care for a patient; bathing a patient; monitoring vital functions; adjusting the ventilator in light of blood gas values.

2. *Guiding another.* The nurse provides direction and guidance to the patient during both phases of deliberate action (intentional and productive). The nurse uses open communication (verbal and nonverbal) to (1) assist the patient in gaining insight into the need for nursing care and the related care measures, (2) guide the patient in exploration of personal valuation of needs for self-care and self-care actions, (3) stimulate motivation, (4) support the patient in actual performance of self-care actions (or dependent care actions), and (5) guide the patient in evaluating desired, expected outcomes.

   EXAMPLES: Assisting a pregnant mother in the selection of foods high in iron; assisting an elder with the use of a walker; assisting a child with crutch-walking; helping a person explore feelings about the decision on elective surgery.

3. *Supporting another.* The nurse assists the patient in carrying out the actions by providing the appropriate physical or emotional support that enables the patient to successfully engage in action and to persevere

until actions achieve the desired, expected outcomes. Reduction of stress and conflict is part of the support rendered.

EXAMPLES: Providing the right supplies at the appropriate time; encouraging the patient with verbal praise and feedback; assisting the patient to walk in the hallway using a gait belt; remaining present with the patient when the doctor conveys the prognosis/diagnosis.

4. *Providing a developmental environment.* The nurse assists the patient in performance of a task or in the achievement of a requisite by altering the conditions associated with or affecting task performance; conditions could involve external factors (environmental or social) or internal factors (physiological or psychological).

EXAMPLES: Following mastectomy, assisting the woman in combing her hair and applying makeup before visiting hours; informing a patient about a support group for postmastectomy patients; attending to the patient's pain before beginning teaching; providing privacy; assisting a mother who is exploring day care resources for her other children so she can spend more time with her hospitalized child.

5. *Teaching another.* The nurse employs appropriate teaching-learning principles to develop knowledge, skills, or motivation in the patient.

EXAMPLES: Teaching a patient about the ostomy and discussing anticipated lifestyle changes because of an ostomy; teaching an older adult safe ways in which to monitor and take multiple medications daily; assisting the patient in problem-solving; assisting a new mother with breast-feeding her first baby.

Nursing Situation

A **nursing** (or health care) **situation** exists when nurses enter into nursing relationships with patients. In the situation the nurse provides and the patient receives nursing care. Orem (1995, p. 134) stated that there are several classifications of nursing situations and argued that classifications vary according to the type of descriptive or characteristic factor used. Different factors used in classifications systems include (1) the complexities of the needs of patients (as in rehabilitation, medical intensive care, surgical intensive care, outpatient surgery, inpatient surgery); (2) the complexities of the need for nursing care (as in intensive care, acute care, home care); and (3) the intended health goals (health promotion, illness prevention). Classifications of nursing situations might employ any combination of factors, such as patient's age, the place of service, and the unit of service. Neonatal intensive care, pediatric intensive care, and adult intensive care are examples of the factor of age being combined with the factor of complexity of required nursing or medical care.

Consistent with the view of nursing as one of the health services, Orem (1995, p. 134) suggested a preferable means of classifying nursing situations in which nurses and patients interact. Health dimensions specify classifications according to health focus. In a classification system based on the health focus, the following characteristic classifying factors are considered: (1) the presence or absence of health deviation(s), (2) the characteristics and values of the health state, and (3) the orientation of life cycle. This classification system will "indicate appropriate health care goals, specify the kinds of health care required, and may also indicate the kinds of obstacles to self-care that are present or could be present" (Orem, 1995, p. 134). Using these factors for a classification system establishes a health care focus for each nursing situation. Health state is a major consideration within this classification system. The definition of health state is "an expressed formulation of an assessment of whether or not the anatomic features and the functioning of individuals is within or outside established norms for individuals of particular ages in particular developmental stages" (Orem, 1995, p. 206). Health state is both a condition and a basic condition factor (see Chapter 3).

The classification system for nursing situations described by Orem (1995, pp. 133-134) incorporates both the health care focus and health state. Orem (1995, p. 134) stated that these were health care situations and that the classification system could be useful to many health care professions. When of concern to nurses, these health care situations are nursing situations. In this text the phrase *nursing situations* will be used.

According to the classification system described by Orem, there are seven nursing situations (Orem, 1995, pp. 134-142):

Group 1: Health Promotion Throughout the Life Cycle

In general, there is absence of health deviation so the health care focus is on health promotion and maintenance and on protection from illness or injury. Actions are directed toward meeting universal and developmental self-care requisites. For each stage of the life cycle, concerns of health promotion and prevention of illness centers on the major events/conditions associated with that stage or in anticipation of the next stage. The general quality of the health state is good to excellent.

Group 2: Recovery

The health care focus is on recovery from a specific health deviation whereby the outcomes of the health deviation and the medical treatment are in curative or regulative modes. Recovery may be very short and simple as in following a case of flu or appendicitis, or recovery may be more complex and require more time as in joint replacement surgery. While a period of care and treatment may extend over time, the expectation is that health deviation will not persist. The overall quality of the health state is generally good.

Group 3: Illness of Undetermined Origin

As the specific type or kind of health deviation(s) is(are) unknown, the health care focus centers around the signs and symptoms of the health deviation(s) and on the diagnostic procedures or techniques employed. Psychological and emotional stress and reaction are important considerations. The perceived threat of the diagnoses proposed as possible explanations of illness influence the degree and extent of psychological and emotional distress. Some persons evidence clusters of symptoms for which no known or determined explanation exists. The quality of the health state can range from serious to mildly ill, although generally, it is good to fair.

Group 4: Genetic and Developmental Defects and Biological Immaturity

The nature of the health deviation addressed is structural or functional problems derived from (1) either genetic/congenital or biological immaturity of bodily systems or (2) the diagnosis or treatment of such health deviations. Persons may experience one health deviation or multiple, as in the child born with multiple defects. Associated health deviations' onset of overt symptoms may not occur until later in life, for example, the person with a structural defect in the heart that is not detected until playing college basketball. Nursing care associated with health deviations of this nature could require short-term intervention (e.g., the child with pyloric stenosis) or could demand lifelong intervention (e.g., the child with spastic cerebral palsy). The quality of the health state may range from mildly to severely ill.

Group 5: Cure or Regulation

The focus of care is on the active cure or regulation of health deviations of determined origins not present at birth. The extent of involvement depends on the nature and severity of the identified health deviation. Health states vary vastly because of the vast number of simple to complex health deviations associated with illness, injury, defect, and disability; also persons frequently experience multiple health deviations at any one time. The nature of the health deviation can be stable or unstable, reflected in observed or anticipated changes over time. For example, a person with well-controlled diabetes is fairly stable with ongoing regulation of the diet, insulin, and exercise. However, a person with very "brittle" diabetes experiences frequent instability. Another factor that influences the stability of the health state is the occurrence of additional health deviations. For example, the person with diabetes has the flu or develops congestive heart failure or high blood pressure. The quality of the health state can range from mildly ill to seriously ill, but it may fluctuate, particularly when the status of the health deviation fluctuates.

Group 6: Stabilization of Integrated Functioning

The focus of care is to stabilize, regulate, and restore vital processes of human functioning. The nature of the health deviations is usually severe, highly unstable, multiple, and complex. Because of the unstable nature of the health state, immediate, persistent, and intense observation and interventions are necessary. Ideally, stabilization of the patient's condition occurs within a short period of time and the patient's status can be "downgraded" to a nursing situation of less intensity, for example, to cure and regulation or even to recovery. In severe cases, the quality of sustained life becomes a major concern. The health state is seriously ill.

Group 7: Terminal Illness

The focus of care is to eliminate, control, or mitigate the effects of or symptoms of health deviations that have severely impaired the vital and functional integrity of the individual, as in the final stages of illness or injury. Concern centers on the physical, psychological, and emotional support. Actions must help patients approach the end of their lives with a sense of control, dignity, and security. The health state is generally poor.

• • •

Use of health care focus as a central classifying factor helps nurses determine and attend to the kinds of health goals intended, the kinds of health care required, and obstacles or potential obstacles to self-care (Orem, 1995, p. 134). Determination of nursing care needs depends on the nurse's ability to assess therapeutic self-care demand and self-care agency and their relationships. Nursing situations classified by health care focus facilitate examination of therapeutic self-care demand. The health care focus of the first nursing situation focuses only on the universal and developmental self-care requisites. Health deviation self-care requisites are added to the universal and developmental self-care requisites in the remaining six nursing situations (Orem, 1995, p. 135). "The linking of the helping and health [care] focuses in nursing practice is mediated by patient variables, therapeutic self-care demand and self-care agency, and the relationship between them" (Orem, 1995, p. 135).

Summary

Basic conditioning factors modify or affect all persons. These basic conditioning factors are applicable to the persons who are the nurses (nurse agents) and their abilities to nurse (nursing agency). The modifying effects of basic conditioning factors on nurse agents validate the uniqueness of each individual nurse. Assessing relevant basic conditioning factors helps to describe and characterize persons who are nurses.

To accomplish the work of nursing, the nurses must exercise nursing agency (that is, activate and employ abilities to nurse). Development of nursing agency occurs via nursing education (basic, advanced, or continuing) and practical experiences of nursing. Exercise of nursing agency takes place in nursing situations. Initial nursing actions require those nursing abilities that focus on determining the current and the projected system of self-care/dependent care, therapeutic self-care demand of the self-care agent or dependent care recipient, abilities of self-care agency or dependent care agency relevant to the demand for care, and the relationship between therapeutic self-care demand and self-care (or dependent care) agency. Factors that influence therapeutic self-care demand and self-care (or dependent care) agency (basic conditioning factors) are considered in the assessments that are part of estimative operations. The transitional operations of nursing culminate in the identification of self-care (or dependent care) deficits.

Nurses seek to identify which persons are in need for nursing care. Nurses employ knowledge and skills to identify patients for whom self-care agency (or in dependent care, combined self-care agency and dependent care agency) is inadequate to meet the needs expressed by therapeutic self-care demand. In these patients self-care or dependent care deficits exist, and when health related or health derived, they are of concern to nursing. Persons with self-care deficits (or dependent care deficits) are the legitimate patients of nursing. Nurses target these self-care and dependent care deficits in their efforts to assist patients in achieving therapeutic self-care or dependent care. Based on knowledge about patients and their existing and projected self-care (or dependent care) deficits, nurses can determine what form nursing must take to help those patients. Nursing actions selected address resolution of the deficit by augmenting, developing, or aiding the exercise of agency or by decreasing the demand.

The basic framework for the delivery of nursing care is evident in the design of the nursing system. A nursing system is the entire system of nursing actions, including those associated with the social, interpersonal, and professional-technological components of the process of nursing. A nursing system delineates (1) the role(s) and responsibilities of the nurse; (2) the role(s) and responsibilities of the patient; (3) the methods of helping leading to specific ordered, sequential nursing actions, which, when produced, will result in nursing care. The overall goal of nursing is to ensure accomplishment of therapeutic self-care (dependent care). Based on the prescribed roles and actions for both nurse and patient, the nursing system may be either supportive-educative, partly compensatory, or wholly compensatory.

Figure 21 and 22 present conceptual framework models for self-care deficit theory of nursing (SCDTN). Figure 21 presents a conceptual model linking the variables of nurse and nursing agency to the variables of the

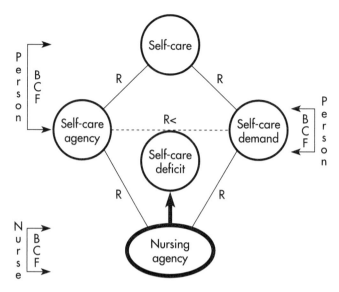

FIGURE 21

Conceptual framework for self-care deficit theory of nursing (SCDTN), pertaining to self-care. *BCFs* = Basic conditioning factors; *R* = relationship; < = deficit relationship. (Modified with permission from Orem, D. [1995]. *Nursing: Concepts of practice* [5th ed., p. 435]. St. Louis, MO: Mosby.)

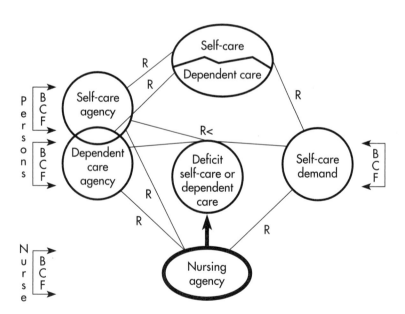

FIGURE 22

Conceptual framework for self-care deficit theory of nursing (SCDTN), pertaining to situations of dependent care. *BCFs* = Basic conditioning factors; *R* = relationship; < = deficit relationship. (Modified with permission from Orem, D. [1995]. *Nursing: Concepts of practice* [5th ed., p. 435]. St. Louis, MO: Mosby.)

self-care system: self-care, therapeutic self care demand, self-care agency, basic conditioning factors, and self-care deficits. Figure 22 presents a conceptual model linking the variables of nurse and nursing agency to the variables of the dependent care system: self-care and dependent care, therapeutic self-care demand, self-care agency and dependent care agency, basic conditioning factors, and self-care and dependent care deficits. The model pertaining to dependent care clearly indicates the complexity of relationships among conceptual elements.

Process of Nursing and Nursing Process

Nursing is deliberate action. Actions associated with and derived from the nursing process evidence a conscious, purposeful selection of activities directed toward identifying and meeting the need for nursing care. The performance of nursing actions results in the production of nursing care. The nurse must always keep in mind that the overall goal of nursing according to self-care deficit theory of nursing (SCDTN; Orem, 1995, pp. 316, 332) is to ensure the accomplishment of therapeutic self-care by doing the following:

- Assisting the patient to become more independent in the performance of self-care (dependent care); patients are assisted in the following:
  1. The *learning* of new self-care (dependent care) abilities (i.e., develop self-care agency or dependent care agency, respectively)

  OR

  2. The *mobilization* of new and current self-care (or dependent care) abilities not previously used (i.e., exercise of self-care agency or dependent-care agency, respectively)
- Assisting in the performance of self-care (or dependent care) actions when interruptions in self-care occur or when self care (or dependent care) abilities decline; patients are assisted by the following:
  1. Having some or all self care (or dependent care) actions *performed* for them
  2. Having some or all self-care (or dependent care) decisions *made* for them

  AND/OR

  3. Having current self care agency (or dependent care agency) protected from further decline

The Process of Nursing

Nursing practice has three component parts: social, interpersonal, and professional-technological (Orem, 1995, pp. 253, 288-290, 302). These three components together represent the entirety of the **process of nursing.** The social, interpersonal, and professional-technological components are interlocking and interdependent. All three occur simultaneously and result in nursing practice. The social and interpersonal components of nursing practice establish the context of nursing situations in which nursing actions of the professional-technological component will occur. Each component has its own technologies (i.e., knowledge associated with skills). Following is a discussion of each of the three components. Figure 23 illustrates the relationships of one component to another and key elements of each component.

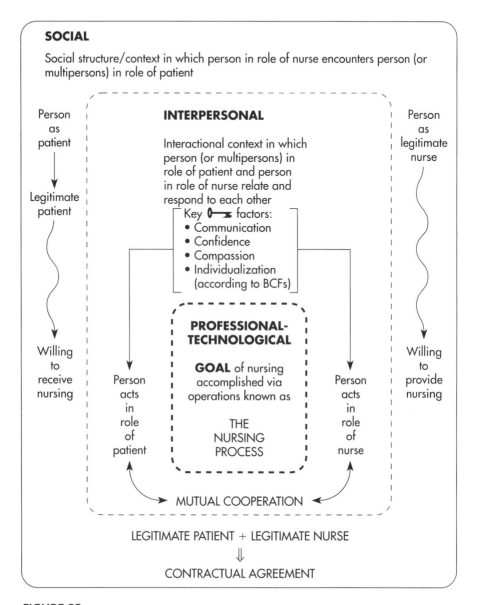

FIGURE 23

Key elements of the social, interpersonal, and professional-technological components of the process of nursing.

Social Component

The **social component** encompasses the nature of nursing as a social institution within society. In the socially defined and sanctioned institution of nursing, both the patient and the nurse have socially defined roles. Two important points address the roles of each:

1. Acceptability of the person as one in need of help is socially defined. Persons best served by nursing are those who truly have a need for nursing care. In self-care deficit theory of nursing, persons with existing or projected self-care deficits (or dependent care deficits) are legitimate patients of nursing. Although the patient remains a participant in self-care as much as possible, the role of the patient in relationship to nursing is fundamentally that of recipient of nursing care (i.e., patient) (Orem, 1995, p. 42). An essential characteristic is that the patient is open and willing to receive nursing care. The type and amount of nursing care needed by the patient varies with time.

2. Various sources provide definitions about what persons can legitimately occupy the role of nurse. Obviously, support for who can rightly and legitimately occupy the role of the nurse is found in regulations and definitions of nursing. These are most readily found in legal statutes about nursing, frequently known as nurse practice acts. Professional definitions endorsed by professional nursing organizations help articulate who nurses are and provide important information about the boundaries of nursing as a helping service. These are important especially as they often address nursing's relationship with other helping professions. Examples of these include those in publications of the National League for Nursing, International Council for Nursing (ICN), and the American Nurses Association (ANA), particularly ANA document *Nursing: A social policy statement* (American Nurses Association, 1980). Nursing education affords one of the first validations of the legitimacy of persons occupying the role of nurse. The person in the role of nurse is in possession of capabilities to nurse learned via specialized education. Before writing licensure examinations, nurses must first graduate from an approved school of nursing. Postbaccalaureate nursing programs provide further credentials for various nursing roles helping to validate those who can legitimately occupy those roles.

   Besides educational and legal criteria, the field of practice or the employer may provide other validations. Professional organizations specific to certain practice areas (such as nurse midwifery and pediatric nurse practitioners) may have specific stipulations about those who qualify for these specialized professional nursing roles. Employment in the role of a registered nurse conveys specific status and authority.

For nursing to occur, a relationship must be established between the person(s) in the role of patient and the person in the role of nurse. The nature of this relationship in the social component is *contractual*. In the contractual agreement, there is a willingness and acceptance on the part of the patient to "receive" nursing care and on the part of the nurse to "give" nursing care. This relationship is essential as nursing can only occur in this interpersonal context. For persons who are unconscious or severely ill, their agreement in the contractual relationship is implicit on entry in the health care facility or institution.

In addition to socially delineated and acceptable roles, the social component of the process of nursing recognizes that nursing occurs in varied socially defined settings within the health care system. In the health care system, roles and relationships among members of the helping professions are defined by the boundaries of each profession. Definitions of roles and responsibilities of patients and nurses are evident in the literature related to health care.

Interpersonal Component

The **interpersonal component** encompasses the nature of the reciprocal person-to-person relationship (i.e., interpersonal) that exists in nursing situations. Within interactions between nurse and patient, the actions of the individual are consistent with the person's role (i.e., one *acts* in the role of patient and the other *acts* in the role of nurse). In the interaction, the intent is that nursing helps the patient by assisting the patient in overcoming self-care (dependent care) limitations associated with self-care deficits or in compensating for these self-care (dependent care) limitations. To accomplish this, the patient-nurse interpersonal interaction is one of *cooperation*. Acknowledgment of the importance and uniqueness of each individual is essential for establishing quality interpersonal relationships. Assessment of basic conditioning factors helps to delineate and describe much of what is unique about the patient and the nurse. Additionally, the patient's family or significant others are other important participants in the interpersonal relationships established in nursing situations. Key factors in interpersonal relationships between patients and nurses are communication, compassion, and confidence. Personality, style of communication, and empathy are also important determinants of the success of interpersonal relationships.

Professional-Technological Component

The **professional-technological component** encompasses all that nurses do for and with patients as they carry out the deliberate actions of nursing. The professional-technological component brings in what nurses do in the context of developing and developed interpersonal relationships. The activities of nurses in this component focus on (1) assisting patients with existing and projected self-care deficits and (2) ultimately, meeting the over-all goal of nursing (i.e., accomplishing therapeutic self-care through regulating the exercise and development of self-care [or dependent care] agency). Thus the patient achieves integrated functioning, health, and well-being.

Orem (1995, pp. 253, 268) stated the professional-technological component focuses on operations that constitute nursing process. Nursing process is the conscious, deliberate, and systematic method of selecting and performing nursing actions and activities that will (1) identify clients who have a need for nursing care (i.e., persons with self-care deficits [or dependent care deficits]), (2) provide and regulate the kind and amount of nursing care needed to assist patients with achieving therapeutic self-care, and (3) lead to formation of appropriate judgments about the effectiveness of the nursing care provided (Orem, 1995, pp. 268-269).

Nursing Process

Meleis (1991, pp. 106-109) stated nursing process is a central concept in the domain of nursing and is often a central concept in many nursing theories. The **nursing process** involves the systematic method of planning and performing nursing care for legitimate patients of nursing (Christensen & Kenney, 1995, pp. 9-12). This systematic methodology uses some problem-solving and decision-making processes combined with applied knowledge to guide nursing practice. Beside the obvious applicability of scientific and empirical knowledge, Firlit (1994, p. 77) suggested that other forms of knowledge such as moral, intuitive, aesthetic, and existential make important contributions to nursing practice and nursing decisions. In the nursing process, the skills of decision-making and problem-solving require a variety of related abilities to be successful, including but not limited to reasoning, understanding, judging, attending, investigating, thinking critically, valuing, planning, acting, performing, and controlling. Using nursing process, nurses will make nursing decisions regarding the following:

- Why a person (or multiperson unit) has a need for nursing care.
- What kind of nursing care is required.
- What the role of the patient and the role of the nurse will be.
- What duration of time nursing care will be required.

Nursing process involves sequential steps in a problem-solving decision-making approach. Different authors describe as few as three steps and some, as many as five. However, Yura and Walsh (1988) have set the "gold standard" with a process that has the following four-step process: (1) assessment and diagnosis, (2) planning, (3) implementation, and (4) evaluation. These four steps of the nursing process can be found in almost every nursing text. Because this four-step approach is so common and because it is a general formula not tied to one nursing theory or model, the term *generic* is used for this approach to nursing process. The steps occur in sequence, but the nursing process is not linear.

Orem's Conceptualization of Nursing Process

According to Orem (1995, pp. 316, 323), nursing must be intentionally designed, constructed, and produced to meet the goal of nursing. Orem (1995) defines nursing process as "nurses' performance of the professional-technologic operations of nursing practice . . . [and] constituted from the nurses' performance of diagnostic, prescriptive, and regulatory or treatment operations with associated control operations including evaluation" (p. 268). She further conceptualizes nursing process as incorporating the concepts derived from the three articulating theories in self-care deficit theory of nursing (SCDTN), particularly the patient variables of therapeutic self-care demand and self-care agency (dependent care agency). Decision-making and problem-solving skills and the related abilities mentioned above are all important in each step as nurses employ nursing knowledge to make sound nursing decisions.

All the abilities related to the performance of the nursing process are essential skills associated with the estimative, transitional, and productive operations of nursing as deliberate action (see Figure 24). Specialized learning, nursing education, is the means of developing abilities that are used by nurses in planning and producing nursing. The collective set of abilities to nurse constitutes nursing agency. When persons who perform nursing (i.e., nurse agents) exercise nursing agency, the result is the production of nursing care.

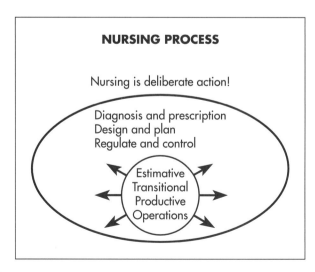

FIGURE 24

Nursing as deliberate action.

The three steps in Orem's nursing process follow (Orem, 1995, p. 268):

Step I: Diagnosis and prescription
Step II: Design and plan
Step III: Regulate and control

A comparison of the steps of the "generic" nursing process (Yura & Walsh, 1988) and Orem's steps of the nursing process is presented in Table 6. Orem (1995, p. 269) agreed with the "generic" approach in that the steps of the nursing process are sequential but the process is not linear. The following discussion expands on each of the three steps of Orem's nursing process.

Step I: Diagnosis and Prescription. Nursing process occurs within the framework established by the social and interpersonal components of nursing practice (Orem, 1995, p. 269). This means that the nurse and patient have a contractual agreement to each function in his or her role (i.e., that of nurse and patient, respectively). In addition, an interpersonal relationship between patient and nurse establishes a system of interaction based on mutual cooperation (Orem, 1995, p. 269). (See the discussion of process of nursing at the beginning of this chapter.)

This first step of the nursing process is diagnosis and prescription, two separate but related tasks (Orem, 1995, pp. 268, 270-273). In this first step, the nurse collects and analyzes data about the patient. Initially, the nurse must establish an appropriate database on which to make the appropriate decisions and judgments as to why a person has a need for nursing care. In this endeavor, the nurse exercises both practical and intellectual processes. This simply means that the nurse collects data by practical processes such as interviewing, taking vital signs, physical examination, and reviewing medical information. The information gathered increases the nursing judgment about the patient variables of therapeutic self-care demand and self-care agency (both as modified by the basic conditioning factors). Additionally, analysis and organization of information and determinations of the need for additional data involve intellectual processes.

TABLE 6 Comparison of Steps in "Generic" Nursing Process to Steps in Nursing Process in Self-Care Deficit Theory of Nursing (SCDTN)	
Generic Nursing Process	**SCDTN Nursing Process**
I. Assessment and diagnosis	I. Diagnosis and prescription
II. Planning	II. Design and plan
III. Implementation	III. Regulate and control
IV. Evaluation	

The collected database represents the information on which the nurse will make judgments (i.e., **nursing diagnoses**). The questions posed in Table 7 represent an outline of this database. Evident from the questions posed in Table 7, the first step involves (1) assessment of the self-care agent in light of basic conditioning factors, (2) determination of therapeutic self-care demand and analysis of self-care agency, (3) identification of self-care deficits expressed as nursing diagnosis statements. Information in response to each question contributes to a judgment made in this first step of the nursing process.

The first step of the nursing process begins with establishment of the contractual and cooperative relationships of the social and interpersonal components of the process of nursing. Data collection, usually prioritized and organized around the basic conditioning factors is the starting point. The outcome of the first step of the nursing process is the identification (or not)

TABLE 7 Assessments and Judgments Made in First Step of Nursing Process Address Essential Questions

Question	Judgment
What are the basic conditioning factors as they exist in the situation for this patient?	Assessment of data regarding self-care agent (SCA)
What are the existing self-care requisites as particularized for this patient?	Assessment of therapeutic self-care demand (TSCD)
What are the self-care actions validly and reliably necessary to meet those particularized self-care requisites?	Calculation of therapeutic self-care demand (TSCD)
What order, organization, and prioritization should be given to the self-care requisites: (a) As viewed by the patient? (b) As viewed by the nurse?	Calculation and prescription of therapeutic self-care demand (TSCD)
What are those self-care (or dependent care) actions valued by the patient as evidenced by the self-care (or dependent care) actions in which the patient engages?	Assessment of self-care agency (SCA) (or dependent care agency [DCA])
What are the self-care abilities (or dependent care abilities) (e.g., knowledge, skills, willingness) of the patient for meeting existing or projected self-care requisites?	Assessment of self-care agency (SCA) (or dependent care agency [DCA])
What are the existing or projected self-care limitations in self-care agency for deliberate action aimed at self-care; what is the adequacy of self-care agency (or dependent care agency)?	Assessment of self-care agency (SCA) (or dependent care agency [DCA])
What, then, are the nursing diagnosis statements that express the self-care (dependent care) deficits that need to be addressed by nursing care?	Determination of self-care (dependent care) deficits leading to formulation of nursing diagnosis statements

EXERCISE

Concepts in Step I of Nursing Process

Test your understanding of the relationships of theoretical concepts in the first step of the nursing process by completing the following statements, filling in the blanks with the correct term.

1. Information about the person performing self-care is sought. This means the nurse assesses the self-care _____. In the case of dependent care, nurses must gather information about both the persons involved in the care system. This means the nurse assesses both the dependent care _____ (who is also the self-care agent) and dependent care _____ is sought.

2. Assessments of the unique individual person's characteristics can be organized according to the framework by the _____.

3. Based on the information obtained, the nurse particularizes the patient's self-care requisites. This means that the nurse calculates the patient's _____.

4. Based on information obtained and in relation to the identified needs for self-care requisites, the nurse assesses the patient's abilities for self-care (or dependent care). This means the nurse assesses the patient's self-care _____.

5. The nurse must at all times consider how all the above are constantly and continuously modified by the _____.

6. Once the nurse has collected and evaluated the data (the self-care requisites and the self-care agency), the presence of either existing or projected self-care deficits (or dependent care deficits) are determined based on the relationship between _____ and _____.

of self-care (dependent care) deficits. Nursing diagnosis statements are expressions of self-care (dependent care) deficits. Nursing diagnoses set the prescriptive framework for the need for nursing care (i.e., prescriptions concerning type, amount, and duration).

The following discussion provides further examination of the components of the first step of the nursing process. This includes a discussion of the approaches nurses use in meeting responsibilities for diagnosis and prescription.

Assessment of Self-Care Agent. The first step of any problem-solving process is to collect and analyze data about the situation or problem. In nursing, the primary concern is the patient or potential patient and that patient's actual or potential need for nursing care. An organizing framework for assessing the uniqueness of each individual helps to assure that the assessment is comprehensive and thorough. One framework derived from the theory is that of the basic conditioning factors. (See Table 1 in Chapter 3.) If the contact with the patient is of greater length and duration, assessment of basic conditioning factors is more detailed with greater depth. In rapidly changing nursing situations or in nursing situations of short duration, assessment of basic conditioning factors proceeds on a priority basis. Orem identified age, developmental state, and health state as three of the most critical for nurses to investigate (Orem, 1995, p. 332).

Beside basic conditioning factors, the patient's perception of health state is another aspect of this part of the assessment. In many texts, this is the patient's "presenting problem." Presenting problems generally refer to the problems or cluster of problems that represent a change in health state or perceived change in health state. This change causes the patient to seek assistance and access the health care system. Examples of this include persistent headaches, trauma from an accident, or just a general feeling of ill-being. Assessments involve more than just identifying the problem from the perspective of signs or symptoms. An important aspect of assessment of self-care agent is identifying the patient's perception of the meaning and impact of the problem(s).

Calculation of Therapeutic Self-Care Demand. Particularization of the needs for self-care and the related care measures (i.e., self-care requisites) is a major activity of nurses in relation to the concept of therapeutic self-care demand. Nurses must validate whether their assessment and prioritization of self-care requisites are consistent with those of their patients. Refer to the sections in Chapter 4 regarding self-care requisites and calculation of therapeutic self-care demand. Activities center around particularization of all self-care requisites and validating which self-care requisites the patient meets without difficulty. See the discussion of composing particularized self-care requisite statements in Chapter 4.

Assessment of Self-Care Agency. Assessment of self-care agency involves the identification and examination of the type, quality, and quantity of those abilities for self-care. The assessment of self-care agency involves an assessment of both the form and content of self-care agency. To review:

- The *form* of self-care agency rests in the foundational capabilities and dispositions, power components, and abilities related to the three self-care operations of deliberate action that are the operations: estimative, transitional, and productive.

- The *content* of self-care agency is made up of the purposes toward which abilities are directed: the self-care requisites.

Assessment of self-care agency has two parts. The first part of assessment focuses on examination and exploration of foundational human abilities and power components. The second part of assessment focuses on examination and determination of those specific abilities associated with the estimative, transitional, and productive self-care operations. Therefore, a two-step approach to the assessment of self-care agency is proposed. The process is investigative. This two-step approach is described below with questions intended to illustrate the inquiry (not meant to be all-inclusive):

Step 1. Initially, certain foundational human abilities (see p. 66) must be addressed with regards to assessment of self-care agency. This aspect addresses questions regarding foundational human abilities which are not only elemental but also pervasive to the functional level of any other abilities that may exist in agency. These foundational human abilities include questions related to the capacities of agency (Orem, 1995, pp. 217-222; Orem, 1979, pp. 210-218; Backscheider, 1974) such as:

- What is the person's capacity for sensation (linked to the five senses and perception)? What is the person's capacity to communicate?
- What is the person's capacity for attending, storing, and processing information and to exercise reason?
- What is the person's capacity for self-examination and self-awareness with regard to self, environment, and motivation?

Step 2. Once the nurse has initially assessed the foundational human abilities of agency, assessment of self-care agency necessitates looking at those specific abilities associated with the estimative, transitional, and productive self-care operations linked to the self-care actions prescribed by each particularized self-care requisite in the calculated therapeutic self-care demand. In relation to each of the self-care operations, assessment leads to identification of abilities and limitations of knowing, judging and decision-making, and engaging in result-achieving actions (see Tables 3 and 4, pp. 69-70, 74). The following format suggests a guide for gathering information in relation to each particularized self-care requisite about abilities related to the three self-care operations for each particularized self-care requisite.

- Abilities associated with estimative self-care operation
  1 In regard to *knowing,* what is the person's ability to accomplish the following?
    a Determine and analyze the meaning and value of (1) the self-care requisites and attending to self-care as it has been and as it should be and (2) the outcome of self-care

      b Determine the relationship between what needs to be done for therapeutic self-care and self-care as it is currently and as it should be

  2 In regard to *result-achieving actions,* what is the person's ability to accomplish the following?

      a Actively seek out information regarding existing and projected self-care requisites

      b Actively seek out information regarding the types of actions necessary to accomplish self-care in the conditions that prevail

- Abilities associated with transitional self-care operation

  1 In regard to *knowing,* what is the person's ability to accomplish the following?

      a Ascribe value and meaning to the alternate self-care actions

      b Reflect on which self-care actions should or should not be done

      c Identify what varied resources are necessary to carry out the alternate self-care actions identified

  2 In regards to *judging and decision-making,* what is the person's ability to accomplish the following?

      a Knowledgeably select those self-care actions that will be effective and therapeutic

      b Set a level of willingness to engage in the required self-care actions

- Abilities associated with productive self-care operation

  1 In regard to *knowing,* what is the person's ability to accomplish the following?

      a Know what the desired or undesirable outcomes are and how to monitor for them

      b Gather and reflect on information resulting from the performance of selected self-care actions

  2 In regard to *judging and decision-making,* what is the person's ability to determine if the self-care actions should be continued, altered, or discontinued?

  3 In regard to *result-achieving action,* what is the person's ability to accomplish the following?

      a Engage in psychomotor skills that require physical movement and manipulation, as necessary to the specified skill of self-care action, and to monitor results of self-care action

      b Gather, locate, and use the resources necessary to the performance of self-care action

On completion of the assessment of abilities for each of the particularized self-care requisites of therapeutic self-care demand, the nurse concludes the assessment of self-care agency by making judgments regarding the *adequacy* of the assessed abilities to meet the particularized self-care requisites. Judgments about presence of self-care limitations contribute to decisions about adequacy. This highly important judgment by the nurse considers not only whether the patient has the necessary self-care abilities, but also whether the patient currently exercises any or all existing abilities (i.e., operability). Nursing judgments regarding the operability and adequacy of self-care agency are essential precursors to the identification of self-care deficits (Orem, 1995, pp. 214, 235-236).

Determination of Self-Care Deficits. The existence of health-derived or health-related self-care deficits justify the patient's need for nursing care. Self-care deficits are identified based on the relationship between therapeutic self-care demand and self-care agency. Whether existing or projected, self-care deficits point out self-care limitations that prohibit the patient from meeting/achieving therapeutic self-care. Self-care limitations are expressions that identify that which restricts or prohibits the patient from performing self-care actions as required to meet needs for self-care. Limitations in self-care abilities or absence of self-care abilities associated with the estimative, transitional, and productive self-care operations result in self-care limitations when those self-care abilities are necessary for the meeting of the self-care requisite.

When self-care abilities are lacking or limited, certain questions must be addressed by the nurse to delineate specifics regarding the patient's need for nursing care. Analysis of the self-care deficit should include answers to the following questions:

- What self-care limitations does the self-care deficit pose?
- Why do these self-care limitations exist?
- Are there any factors that would necessitate the patient refraining in exercising self-care abilities (i.e., should the patient be encouraged in performing or participating in self-care or not)?
- Are there any factors that would necessitate protection of the patient's abilities from further harm or decline?
- What is the patient's future potential for engaging in self-care (i.e., what are realistic goals about the patient's involvement in self-care)?

The same process of assessment discussed here applies, in parallel, to assessment of dependent care agency.

Formulation of Nursing Diagnostic Statements. Once all the above factors have been considered, the nurse can exercise judgment as to patient's need for nursing care based on clearly identified self-care deficits; the need for nursing care is expressed as **nursing diagnosis statements** representing the self-care deficit.

Figure 25 presents a summary of the major actions in the first step of the nursing process.

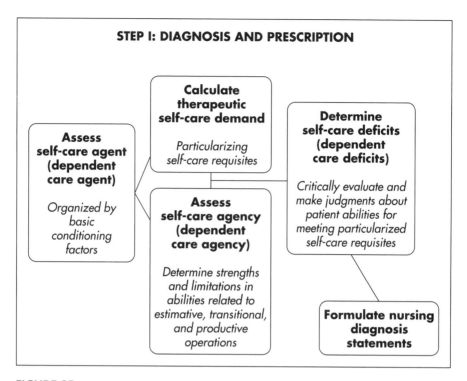

FIGURE 25

Actions in the first step of the nursing process.

Step II: Design and Plan. In the second step of the nursing process, design and plan, the nurse exercises intellectual processes to make nursing decisions pertaining to the type and degree of nursing care needed by the patient (Orem, 1995, pp. 268, 280). First, the nurse reviews the needs for self-care (dependent care) expressed by the therapeutic self-care demand and the self-care (or dependent care) actions necessary for meeting therapeutic self-care demands. Then, the nurse examines the nature of and type of all self-care (dependent care) deficits as expressed in the nursing diagnosis statements. Consideration must be given as to type, amount, and duration of needed nursing care.

Based on this examination, the question the nurse must address at this point is: *"Who can and/or should perform self-care actions [dependent care actions] that require movement in space and controlled manipulation?"* (Orem; 1995, p. 306). The appropriate nursing system is selected based on the answer provided. See the discussion of nursing system in Chapter 5.

The nursing system selected identifies who will be engaged in performing care actions necessary to meet the therapeutic self-care demand (i.e., the performance of actions consistent with the prescribed roles for nurse and patient). The **plan of care,** which follows the selection of nursing system, specifies how and in what way these roles will be enacted to accomplish therapeutic self-care. The plan of care addresses who acts when to perform what care actions in what action sequence in a given setting using what methods and what equipment or resources (see Figure 26).

EXERCISE

Nursing Systems

In the blank on the right, identify the nursing system that corresponds with the three possible answers to the question of who can and should perform self-care actions.

Answer	*Nursing System*
The patient	_____
The patient or the nurse	_____
The nurse	_____

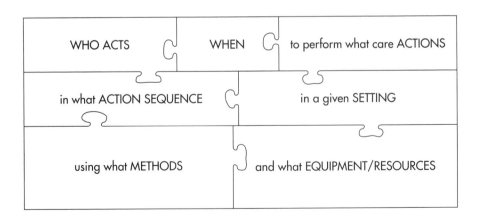

FIGURE 26

Plan: Putting the pieces of the puzzle together in the right way.

The plan of care consists of the following:

- Prescribed patient outcomes (derived from and related to the nursing diagnosis): patient outcomes are expressed in terms that are patient centered and behavioral.
- Accompanying set of "nursing actions" for the stated patient outcome(s):

Characteristics of nursing actions are as follows:

1. Specifically and logically derived from the methods of helping selected
2. Directed toward the patient outcome(s) specified
3. Specific, logically ordered, and sequential actions that prescribe and set forth what actions the nurse and patient will each perform to *cooperatively* regulate and manage self-care
4. Specifications for such things as time, place, environmental conditions, equipment and supplies

Figure 27 presents a summary of the major actions of the second step of the nursing process.

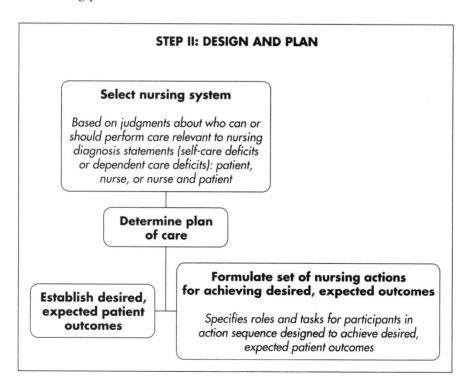

FIGURE 27

Actions of the second step of the nursing process.

Step III: Regulate and Control. In the third step of the nursing process, the nurse exercises both practical and intellectual processes. In the first phase (i.e., regulate) of step III the nurse initiates and carries out the actions specified in the plan of care and in accordance with the selected methods of helping. Care actions are performed by either the nurse or the patient as specified in the plan of care as "nursing actions." The nurse carries out actions appropriate to the methods of helping when providing nursing care for patients. Therefore the actions of the plan are operationalized and nursing care is both produced and managed. The goal is the accomplishment of therapeutic self-care (dependent care).

In the second phase (i.e., control) of this third step, the nurse assesses changes (both internal and external to the patient) and the desired, expected patient outcomes as stated in the plan of care. The nurse exercises knowledge and judgment in determining the sufficiency and efficiency of the planned care actions for (1) meeting therapeutic self-care and (2) exercising, protecting, and developing self-care agency.

Questions addressed in this second phase should include the following:

- Were the nursing actions effective in meeting the patient outcomes established? If not, why not?
- Were the patient outcomes met? If not, why not?
- Were the self-care deficits posed by the nursing diagnosis statement(s) resolved? If not, why not?
- Overall, was the goal/purpose of nursing care accomplished?

Most often data obtained in this phase of the cycle of the nursing process are reentered as new relevant data collected for the diagnosis and prescriptive step; this leads to new conclusions regarding the need for nursing care and the type of nursing care needed. Conclusions regarding the persistence of self-care deficits or the emergence of new self-care deficits indicate a need for continued nursing care. Resolution of self-care deficits indicate that nursing care is no longer needed.

Figure 28 summarizes actions of the third step of the nursing process.

Summary

Nursing, as deliberate action, results when nurses exercise abilities that produce action systems. These action systems assist patients with the intent of assuring the accomplishment of therapeutic self-care (dependent care). Nurses exercise abilities in three components of the process of nursing: social, interpersonal, and professional-technological. The social and interpersonal components set the context for the interactions between nurses and patients. The professional-technological component encompasses all that nurses do for and with patients. The actions of nurses in the professional-technological component are operations that consitute nursing process.

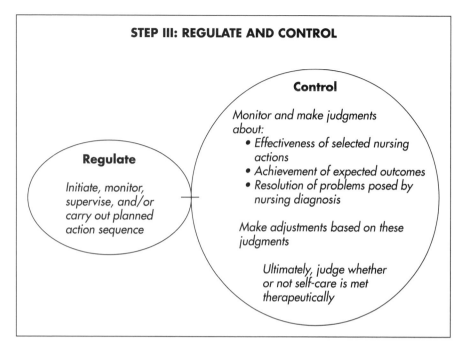

FIGURE 28
Actions of the third step of the nursing process.

Nursing process is a conscious, deliberate, and systematic method of select-ing and performing activities that (1) identify who can benefit from nurs-ing care, (2) identify what kind, type, and amount of nursing care will best assist patients in achieving therapeutic self-care (dependent care) now and in the near future, (3) initiate and sustain the planned nursing care, and (4) judge whether or not nursing care has achieved its intended purpose(s). The three steps of the nursing process as conceptualized by Orem are di-agnosis and prescription, design and plan, and regulate and control.

Operationalizing Orem's Nursing Process

CASE STUDIES

OUTLINE

This chapter presents three case studies. The first case study is a young adult college student whose health state is relatively stable. The health care focus of this case study is on primary prevention and health promotion. The second case study is a dependent care situation involving a young child with a health deviation. The third case study is an older adult experiencing problems associated with the normal aging processes and attempting to manage independent living. The health care focus of both the second and third case studies is on primary and secondary prevention and restorative care and regulation of care, one in the hospital setting and one in the home setting.

The purpose of case studies is to assist students of Orem's theory in (1) exploring and understanding theoretical concepts and (2) developing and exercising nursing abilities related to the nursing process. Case studies afford opportunities for critical thinking and problem-solving in the nursing process. Assessment of the patient (the self-care agent[s]), (and, if applicable, the dependent care agent[s]) is the beginning of the first step of the nursing process. The case studies of this chapter present information about each patient by providing the data for assessment of the self-care agent (and dependent care agent). Basic conditioning factors serve as the organizers for the assessed information about each self-care agent (and in the second case, the dependent care agent). Activities for these case studies center around (1) the completion of the first step of the nursing process, diagnosis and prescription, (2) design and plan for care in the second step of the nursing process, and (3) discussion of regulate and control as the third step of the nursing process.

As in most case studies, client information provided is illustrative and brief. While admittedly brief, cases provide sufficient information for the purposes intended here. Critique and analysis of the case study assessment data of the self-care agent or dependent care agent contribute to developing skills of assessment. Feel free to expand on the case by supplementing further assessment of the agent or agency. The following directions apply to each case study.

Using the pages provided as work templates, document your work in the appropriate columns on the page provided (or make up your own system of documentation).

Directions for Case Studies
Step I: Diagnosis and Prescription

Assessment of the self-care agent (and, if applicable, the dependent care agent) initiates this step of the nursing process. This initial database is the assessment of the self-care agent (with, if applicable, dependent care agent) and is provided by the case study. Basic conditioning factors organize the database as presented. Read the case information provided. Compare the information to the assessment parameters for each of the basic conditioning factors described in Table 1 (see p. 26). Analyze the data in the case with the suggested parameters for assessing basic conditioning factors. What areas are omitted? How would you formulate interview questions to provide the additional data? Are there other sources or means by which information might be gathered? (NOTE: In the second case study for the child, developmental state is left blank so you can explore norms for the chronological age and determine if health deviation has affected development status: read the case for clues.)

Data collection and assessment of individual information about the self-care or dependent care agent are major precursors to calculation of therapeutic self-care demand and assessment of self-care or dependent care agency. Knowledge about the person and relevant basic conditioning factors facilitates identification of particularized self-care requisites important for achieving therapeutic self-care. Remember therapeutic self-care demand focuses on what self-care actions are necessary for the accomplishment of therapeutic self-care. The particularized self-care requisites of therapeutic self-care demand do not address whether or not the self-care agent can or should perform the action. The particularized self-care requisite only addresses the action necessary for the self-care agent's self-care. First, work on particularizing self-care requisites for the universal and developmental self-care requisites; add health deviation self-care requisites if health deviations are present. Identify interrelationships (i.e., articulations) among self-care requisites.

Next, assess self-care agency and determine the assets (abilities) and limitations. Inferences about self-care agency (dependent care agency) must be drawn from the behavioral evidence presented in the case and knowledge of the effects of basic conditioning factors on abilities to perform self-care actions (or dependent care actions). Judgments about the adequacy of self-care agency (or dependent care agency) for meeting the demands set by self-care requisites are important for identification of self-care deficits (dependent care deficits).

Finally, examine the relationship between therapeutic self-care demand and self-care agency and determine if existing or projected self-care deficits are present. For those self-care requisites in which you find agency is insufficient (i.e., inadequate because of undeveloped or inoperable abilities) to meet the therapeutic self-care demands, self-care (or dependent care) deficits serve as the basis for nursing diagnosis statements and legitimize the need for nursing care. State each self-care (or dependent care) deficit as a nursing diagnosis.

STEPS IN OREM'S NURSING PROCESS

STEP I: DIAGNOSIS AND PRESCRIPTION

Therapeutic Self-Care Demand (TSCD)				Self-Care (Dependent Care) Agency (SCA/DCA)				Self-Care Deficits (SCDs) (nursing diagnosis statements)
Particularized Self-Care Requisite (PSCR)	Related SCRs			Abilities	Limitations	Adequacy		
	U	D	HD			Yes	No	

D = Developmental; *HD* = health deviation; *SCR* = self-care requisite; *U* = universal.

Selected Nursing Diagnosis (conclusion of step I)	STEP II: DESIGN AND PLAN A. Indicate type of nursing system under design and give rationale for selection:		STEP III: REGULATE AND CONTROL
	Expected Patient Outcome	B. Plan Plan of Care: Actions and Role Prescriptions	

Step II: Design and Plan

Work in steps II and III of the nursing process is appropriate only when there are existing or projected self-care deficits. Once you have identified existing or projected self-care deficits (or dependent care deficits in the second case study), make your first decision for step II of the nursing process: design and plan. Ask yourself: What is the type of nursing system applicable in this case? Remember, the nursing decision about type of nursing system is not based on a single, selected self-care deficit. Rather, selection of nursing system requires a total view of demands and deficits.

After you have identified the nursing system, select one of the self-care deficits you stated as a nursing diagnosis statement in step I and develop a plan of care. Your plan of care should include expected patient outcomes and a relevant plan of care—specifying care actions and role prescriptions. Make sure that the plan of care is a logically ordered, sequential action system that includes role prescription for the patient (self-care or dependent care agent), nurse, or other care providers (e.g., respiratory therapists, physical or occupational therapists, nurse specialists, social worker, dietitian). The plan of care should include self-care (dependent care) and nursing care actions that aim at continued monitoring of the patient's situation and that focus on changing the current status of the patient. The plan of care should also emphasize the types and amounts of resources that may be necessary for success.

Step III: Regulate and Control

In conclusion, discuss ways in which you would regulate the self-care (dependent care) and nursing care actions proposed in your plan of care. Because this is a paper-and-pencil exercise, actual regulation is not an option. However, you can explore what types of nursing care actions might be needed to manage the action system as an ongoing effort toward therapeutic self-care. How would you monitor the plan of care and the data needed for judgments about adequacy of the nursing system/plan of care?

C A S E   S T U D Y   **1**

Tristen Heart

Age: 19 years, 3 months   **Gender:** Female

Developmental State

T. states that she has several friends in her dormitory including one "new" friend she hopes will become close. Also she has a few close female friends she has known since grade school, but they all live in her hometown and go to different colleges. She states she misses the closeness of these relationships since coming to college. She states she feels like she "gets along well" with her college roommate, stating they met last year as freshmen while taking similar classes as they are pursuing related majors. This is the first they have shared a room. She dated in high school occasionally but not since coming to college; she desires to date. She currently is pursuing career goals by attending a second year of college, majoring in sociology. She is just starting her major and feels, simultaneously, excited and anxious. She states that in talking to lots of people on campus, she has recently expressed concern over career choice. She evidences both concrete and abstract thought patterns, currently doing "B" to "C" work in her major.

Conclusion(s): Young adulthood—Erikson's stage of intimacy versus isolation (Murray & Zentner, 1993): expanding social relationships, comfortable with sense of self, and able to share thoughts and feelings with other(s), looking toward future goals; cognitive, language, and gross/fine motor and psychosocial developmental skills are consistent with chronological age.

Health State

HISTORY

Family: Unremarkable; father has high blood pressure; maternal grandparents died following accident during the first year of her mother's marriage.

Personal: Unremarkable; usual immunizations; T. had chickenpox as small child; she denies asthma, hay fever, etc.; menses occurs every 30 days, regular and moderate flow, of 5 to 6 days duration since age 13.

REVIEW OF SYSTEMS

Subjective: T. doesn't smoke and avoids situations where people are smoking. She has no difficulty breathing and does not become short of breath if she runs up a flight of stairs in the dormitory. She drinks 2 to 3 cans of Diet Pepsi-Free daily and rarely drinks alcohol. She reports "upset" in stom-

CASE   STUDY   **1** — cont'd

ach frequently when studying (this especially when studying before tests or meeting deadlines for papers) and takes Rolaids for "relief."

A 24-hour diet recall follows:

Breakfast:	Toaster Tarts (2)
	Diet Pepsi-Free
Lunch:	T. states she skipped this meal.
Supper:	Macaroni and cheese
	Broccoli
	Strawberry frozen yogurt
	Water and Diet Pepsi-Free
Study snack:	Peanut butter and crackers
	"Few" cookies sent by grandmother

T. states that this recall is typical of how she eats when at college, although she drinks several cups of coffee at night and drinks "lots" of Diet Pepsi-Free. Her weight has increased by about 10 lb since coming to college. She reports feeling really tired lately.

T. reports no difficulty with elimination. She voids 4 to 5 times per day and has a bowel movement every day or every other day. Her last menstrual period was 2 weeks ago, and she denies problems except feeling sensation of "fullness" in the premenstrual phase. She walks to classes and takes tennis in physical education class, which she does not enjoy because it is in the middle of the day. She stays up until midnight or 1 AM almost every night. She has difficulty falling asleep and staying asleep and does not feel rested. She feels like she cannot relax when in bed and is unable to sleep during the day even though she feels tired. T. states she feels positive about friends, although on campus she is not included in all events; at times, she feels left out. She further states she feels uncomfortable when boys talk to her. Lately she has remained more to herself, feeling she wants to go out but that she now should study more because of "C" grades. Generally, she sees herself as careful: she prevents hazards—sees physicians, has immunizations, dresses properly for weather, and exercises care when crossing campus at night (from the library). T. expresses concern that she is not doing as well at college as she would like. She talked to professors about her grades but has only some small progress by getting a few "Bs" with more studying.

Objective: Ht: 5 feet, 1 inch; Wt: 145 lb; T: 37.1° C oral; P 76, apical, NSR; R 16, recovery index normal; BP 126/78

T. appears fatigued and untidy. Overall she is well nourished and well hydrated. Anterior/posterior lungs are clear. Heart rate is strong and regular. Mucous membranes are pink. Capillary refill is brisk. Skin turgor is good. Skin is intact, warm, and dry. T. moves all extremities equally well with good range of motion; she has no problems with gait or balance. T. does not wear either glasses or contact lenses. Other aspects of the physical examination are unremarkable.

Patient's Perception of Health State

T. perceives herself in good health, although she has had trouble lately "enjoying" food and meals and feeling stressed and tired.

Health Deviations

T. reports no illness, injury, or disability at this time.

Sociocultural-Spiritual Orientation/Family System

T. is white and Protestant, stating that church and church school have always been important in her family and home life, but she states she has not found a church "home" since coming to college. She only attends church irregularly while away from home. States that her paternal grandparents lived close to her hometown; her grandmother never worked, but her grandfather is a retired school principal. She often visited these grandparents as a child, sometimes spending her summers with them. She continues to enjoy their attentiveness and encouragement. Her maternal grandparents, immigrants from Germany, are deceased. Both her parents work; one owns a car dealership, and the other works as a nurse. She has one brother, now in high school, and one sister, age 10. Her family lives in the same small town where she grew up. Her home is approximately 3 hours away from campus. T. states that her parents and grandparents believe in the work ethic. Both parents encourage her in her college studies. She currently has a major in sociology.

T. states she was not active in a lot of organizations in high school because she spent most of her time studying. She was proud to be valedictorian of her graduating class. As a result, she was the recipient of several scholarships that help pay her college tuition; maintenance of these scholarships makes studying and grades very important to her. She works at a local (i.e., near home) business during the summers to help with expenses during the school year but is not working while at college. T. states that she has thought about working while at college because she is hoping her parents will help her obtain a car.

Patterns of Living

T. states that she stays up late to study almost every night and that she used to get up early enough to shower, dress, groom, and eat breakfast, but

CASE   STUDY   **1** — cont'd

lately has been skipping breakfast to sleep longer before her first class at 9 AM. Her exercise now consists mainly of walking across campus and tennis classes twice a week; although she states she used to swim or walk at least three times a week. T. keeps some snacks and "food for on-the-run" in dormitory room. She rarely drinks milk. She denies any food allergies. T. states she used to go home more frequently last year but this year has gone home less because she feels too busy. T. states she perceives herself as "basically healthy" and that her last physical examination was for college admission (see also Health State).

Environment (Conditions of Living)

When not in college, T. returns to family home in small town of 4000 in the southern part of the state. She first left there to come to small private university as a freshman. On campus, she currently lives in a fairly modern college coeducational dormitory, sharing a room with a girl who is also a sophomore. Meals are provided through university's food service. She and her roommate share a small refrigerator in their room. Roommate works and often does not eat meals. T. states she has recently begun skipping meals also.

Available Resources

Family: T. has significant others: parents, grandparents, and a few close friends—all in her home town.

Financial: T. receives financial aid and scholarships for college and uses money made during the summer for expenses. Both parents are employed with her mother's job group insurance covering T. as long as she is a full-time student under age 23. She states she does not spend much except for personal items and occasional meals in the campus fast-food cafeteria and is dependent on maintaining scholarships.

Time: T. perceives she does not have much time to study, although she reports studying 48 to 50 hours each week in addition to class time. T. states she feels very busy.

Other: All campus student resources are available to T., including counseling and health services and university food service. T. states that she has health insurance through her mother's employer as long as she is a full-time student. T. has a private physician at home to whom she has gone all her life.

CASE STUDY **1** — cont'd

Health Care System

T. is at the university health service today to get something different to help her "upset stomach," which she sees as a minor problem only because it interferes with her studies. She has seen the university health service nurse for minor illnesses since coming to college. She is aware that the university health service will help students get clinic/physician appointments as needed. A community hospital is located four blocks from campus. She has a private physician in her hometown.

CASE STUDY **2**

Carlos Ramirez

Age: 2 years, 1 month   **Gender:** Male

Developmental State

See Directions for Case Studies, Step I: Diagnosis and Prescription (p. 120), to conduct a developmental assessment.

Health State

HISTORY

Past: C. was born at full-term following an uneventful pregnancy and delivery; his birth weight was 6 lb 3 oz. C.'s mother reports that C. was bottle-fed as were all the other children, reporting that they bought cans of formula as advised in the Women, Infants, and Children (WIC) Clinic. C. is only allowed a bottle at night now. C. has drunk 2% milk and eaten table food for a little more than 1 year. He is current on all immunizations except for his measles-mumps-rubella vaccine. C.'s mother states she took him to the clinic 1 week ago; since he was not well at that time, the measles-mumps-rubella vaccine was postponed. NKA (no known allergies). In a systems review of C.'s history, no prior complications/problems were noted. C.'s mother stated that C. has been very strong and healthy until this present illness.

Present: Until 1 week ago C. was his "normal" self according to C.'s mother and father. Lately he seems to tire easily and takes two naps a day instead of the usual one. When awake, he is more cranky and irritable and

C A S E   S T U D Y   **2** — c o n t ' d

cries more. He continues to spend his days playing in the family apartment; the parents feel he normally acts much more like his older siblings did at the same age although he sucks his thumb and is "always chewing on something." One week ago he started to refuse foods frequently and had two episodes of vomiting not accompanied by diarrhea. He has refused to eat all foods for the last day. The parents brought him to the clinic. From there, he was admitted to the hospital because he had not slept through the last two nights and constantly cries with his knees drawn up slightly. On admission, the following observations were made:

Ht: 33 inches; Wt: 26.5 lb; T 37.0° C; P 120 (crying); R 38 (crying); BP (right arm) 104/64

slight tremoring, irritable and crying; slapping out at nurse and parent when having vitals taken

Patient's Perception of Health State

Patient is anxious and irritable since hospitalization and clings to mother with evident separation anxiety. Because of his age and stage of development, no evident comprehension of health deviation is expected or seen.

Parents are anxious about the child's condition and express concern about other children in family. They told the interpreter and the nurse that they have no previous knowledge of this disease and do not understand that this is "something" that he got by eating the "wrong things."

Health Deviations

At the conclusion of the second hospital day, the diagnosis of lead poisoning (plumbism) was confirmed.

Health Care System

Physician's orders

Orders on admission, completed or in progress:

CBC with differential	Urinalysis, clean catch
Chest x-ray	Chemistry profile
RBC smear	24-hour urine for ALA
Blood screen for lead	X-ray long bones
EP ratio	Abdominal flat plate

Current orders

Regular diet as tolerated	Feosol (start after chelation)
Bedrest with BRP if tolerated	IV D5-.25NS @ 30 ml/hr
Tylenol prn for pain/fever >38.5° C	Strict I & O
Calcium disodium edetate IV	Seizure precautions
BAL IM	VS q4h

C A S E   S T U D Y   **2** — c o n t ' d

Sociocultural-Spiritual Orientation/Family System

C. and his family live in a neighborhood best described as approximately 60% Hispanic where the children have greater English proficiency than parents, unemployment is high and job opportunities are low, and most all dwellings are high-rise, multifamily buildings. C.'s father was injured in a street accident 3 years ago and has a chronic back problem, which makes it difficult for him to find and keep work outside of the home. At this time the father has been unemployed for 3 months, although he actively looks for work during the day. With the loss of that job, the family's medical benefits were also lost. C.'s mother works part-time as a cleaning lady for a firm that cleans office buildings at night. She sleeps during the day and watches the children when her husband goes out to look for work. Two of C.'s older siblings attend the local Head Start program; two (twins) are younger than he. Sibling's ages are 1, 4, and 5. The mother has no nearby relatives, but the father has family nearby. The paternal grandparents live far away in a southern state, and the maternal grandparents live in Mexico. The family attends St. Mary's Church in their neighborhood and sees themselves as active in their faith. C.'s mother has a rosary, which she keeps on his bedside stand now that he is in the hospital. Spanish is the primary language spoken in the home. C.'s father has fairly good English speaking ability and comprehension; the mother's ability is only fair. The father comes to the clinic appointments and hospital to serve as translator for C.'s mother.

Patterns of Living

C. is cared for by both his parents although the mother is the primary caregiver. During the day C. is at home with his mother who dozes between mealtimes. C. and his siblings play within the apartment. The father is, at times, at home to help watch C. and his siblings while the mother sleeps. At night, the father is at home while the mother works, but C. usually sleeps through the night. C. feeds himself but still needs help with dressing. He had been doing well with toilet training but recently has had many "accidents." His mother states that he really does not brush his teeth and that she hopes to get the clinic dentist to see C. soon.

Environment (Conditions of Living)

C. lives in a two-bedroom apartment in a tenement in a large urban setting. The building is in poor condition not having been modernized in the last 30 years. Parents report paint is peeling and numerous holes are found in the plaster work of the walls. The two-bedroom, one-bath apartment houses C., his parents, and his four brothers and sisters. There is a fire escape

CASE   STUDY   **2** — c o n t ' d

outside the main room, which the family uses in the summer when it is hot as there is no air conditioning. Heat is supplied by an old system with a water boiler and radiators; the radiators have been painted several times and give off inconsistent heat in the cold months. At this present time, C. is hospitalized in a four-bed room of the pediatric unit of a large medical center complex.

Available Resources

Family: There are two maternal aunts and one paternal uncle, all with families and children, who live close by in the same neighborhood. There is evidence of mutual family support among these sibling-families.

Environmental resources: The large urban setting in which C. lives provides a wide array of facilities for health care, entertainment, etc. Mass transit subway and bus lines are available. An interpreter is available within hospital and clinic.

Health care resources: C. was seen in a neighborhood clinic that is a satellite to the large medical center in which he is now hospitalized; he is seen by physicians/residents on service. In the clinic the family has been assigned to one nurse but always sees a different physician.

Financial: The source for the family income comes from one part-time job and some unemployment compensation, which will soon run out. There is no insurance for health/illness coverage. Recently C.'s mother received a Medicaid card.

C A S E   S T U D Y   **3**

Clarence Atkins

Age: 72 years   **Gender:** Male

Developmental State

C. is a retired widower. He retired 6 years ago after working for a road construction company for 18 years; he states he worked general "building jobs" here and there before going to work for this company. C. states, "I always did like to build something with my hands." He has several pieces of hand-whittled work in his home. He states, "Things just aren't the way they used to be," noting that he cannot do fine work because of his arthritis, he has to cook for himself now that his wife is gone, and he cannot hear "real good" even though he has "this new-fangled hearing aid." He states that "this getting old is just hell" especially when you feel "kind of helpless" and have to depend on "your kids for help." He states, "Oh well, I can't complain too much, I've lived a good life." C. does like to go to the library but states it is a lengthy bus trip involving one transfer. He finds he is having to make some major adjustments since his wife's death 1 year ago.

Health State

HISTORY

Family: Both his parents, wife, and one son are deceased. His father died in an automobile accident when C. was 10; his mother died of a stroke at the age of 70. C. has eight siblings of which he is the oldest. One sibling died of a heart attack at the age of 69, and all other siblings are alive. One sibling has diabetes. No history of sickle cell trait or disease.

Personal: C. was wounded in the leg when in the army. He broke his arm as a child and his ankle 15 years ago in a work-related accident. At that time he was told his blood pressure was high and has taken medication for this ever since. He has smoked cigarettes since he was 16 and occasionally smokes a "good cigar." He currently smokes only one pack of cigarettes a day, as he has been "cutting back." Four years ago he had a "mild" heart attack and was in the hospital for 5 days.

C A S E   S T U D Y   **3** — c o n t ' d

REVIEW OF SYSTEMS

Subjective:

A 24–hour diet recall follows:

Breakfast: Regular coffee with milk
             Toaster waffles with butter and syrup

Lunch: Cold meat sandwich
             Chicken noodle soup
             Regular coffee with milk

Supper: Ham and beans
             Corn bread with butter
             Regular coffee with milk

Snack: Cookies
             Regular coffee with milk

C. states that this recall is typical of daily diet, as he does not do much cooking. He also states he has recently "been a little off his feed." Reports no difficulty with elimination: urinates five to six times per day ("but not much at one time") and passes soft bowel movement every day because he takes Milk of Magnesia every night. He uses the elevator and rides the city bus. He states he walks for a little while each day in the nearby city park if the weather is good. Has difficulty staying asleep, waking up with a cough and feeling short of breath. He feels rested only because he naps in his recliner.

Objective: Ht: 6 feet, 1 inch; Wt: 210 lb; T 37.1° C oral; P 90, apical, slightly irregular; R 28 somewhat shallow, with rales notable in lower lobes; speech is breathy; BP 160/98

Overall C. appears well-nourished and well-hydrated. He has a slight shuffling gait but fairly good upright posture. There is a slight yellowing to sclera. Mucous membranes are pink and moist. Capillary refill is brisk in upper extremities but prolonged in lower extremities. Lower extremities evidence +1 pitting edema. Skin turgor is good. Skin is intact, warm, and dry; skin is dry and scaly. C. moves all extremities equally well with fair range of motion; however, the joints in C.'s hands are noted to be swollen and tender, slightly hot with diminished range of motion. C. wears glasses and a hearing aid (in right ear).

Patient's Perception of Health State

C. perceives himself as "pretty darn good for my age." Does recognize having trouble with high blood pressure and a little trouble "gettin' 'round and doin' for myself lately." He sees himself as "gettin' by."

C A S E   S T U D Y   **3** — c o n t ' d

Health Deviations

Congestive heart failure
Rheumatoid arthritis
Hypertension

Health Care System

Physician's Orders

Pepcid qd at hs	Procan SR tid
Lanoxin qd in AM	Meclomen tid
Vasotec bid	Lasix qd in AM
Norvasc bid	Mevacor qd with evening meal
K-Dur with food qid	ASA (1 tab) qd

Physician is in a multiphysician corporate clinic. Home health nursing service is scheduled to begin today.

Sociocultural-Spiritual Orientation/Family System

C. is black male widower and retired laborer. C. is a veteran having served in the army right after high school. C.'s wife of 45 years died 1 year ago of a sudden stroke. He states that it took them all by surprise. C. states that the support of his children and his faith were instrumental in coping with this loss. He is a member of a Protestant church, but it is too far from his current residence for him to attend regularly. He has three children: two daughters (ages 39 and 41) and one son (age 44). He states that they had one other son who died at birth. He has a total of seven grandchildren. His older daughter lives in the same community, but his son and other daughter live several hundred miles away. He usually sees them only once a year. His older daughter, who is a divorced, single parent, comes by to help once a week by taking him to the grocery store. This daughter's oldest child recently began driving and has stopped by on occasion.

Patterns of Living

C. usually retires every night after the evening news. He states he sleeps poorly, often waking with a cough and shortness of breath. He is unable to sleep after 6 AM but often naps during the day in his recliner when watching television. He has had dentures for 30 years. He fixes his own meals. His daughter takes him to his doctor appointments. He takes several medications each day. He states he really should do better at taking them all, explaining "There's so many, it can get downright confusing." He states he

C A S E   S T U D Y   **3** — c o n t ' d

used to sometimes "play ball" with his grandson, but that it is getting too hard to bend over and get the ball and also harder to throw the ball.

Environment (Conditions of Living)

C. lives alone is a subsidized housing for older adults. He moved to this location 6 months ago after he and his children "sorted out things" after his wife died. He lives in a small apartment with one bedroom and an efficiency-size kitchen in a 10-story building located in a large rural community (city of 70,000). Built nearly 15 years ago, this was the only residential building constructed in an urban renewal effort. There is an elevator in the building and laundry facilities in the basement. Residents are discouraged from having their own washers and dryers in their apartments. The operation of the building comes under the city's public housing authority. Most of the shopping has moved to the farther east side of the town, and "downtown" businesses once located near this building have faded away or moved to other locations. There is a city bus service stop at the front entrance of the building.

Available Resources

Family: One daughter and grandchild close by who assist by visiting and taking him to appointments and shopping. Frequent contact with other children by phone. The son pays for the phone service.

Financial: C. has a small pension from his company's retirement plan. However, as he only came to this company late in his working life and had no other retirement plans, his pension is small. This company did not offer retirement health care coverage. He also receives a Social Security check once a month. He has Medicare for health care costs but no other supplemental insurance. He is thankful that they had a small insurance policy for his wife that covered most of the funeral costs.

Time: C. states he has time "on his hands."

Other: A senior citizen center is located in the community. The local parks and recreation department plans activities for senior citizens at the community center. The public housing authority provides for senior services within the retirement building. Home care/health nurse is scheduled to begin seeing C. today.

Summary

Work with case studies presented in this chapter offers opportunities to apply the concepts of Orem's self-care deficit theory of nursing within the nursing process as conceptualized by Orem (1995, pp. 268-284). Each case presents a different patient, setting, and health care focus. Data about patients in each case are presented and organized according to basic conditioning factors. The first case deals with an individual young adult patient who is in a good-to-excellent health state; the health care focus suggests a need for primary prevention and health promotion. The second case presents a patient who is a dependent care recipient and dependent care agent dyad (in this case a child-parent dyad). The child's health is good to fair; and the health care focus suggests a need for curative and regulatory care and health promotion. The third case deals with an individual older adult patient whose health state is fair with several health deviations. The health care focus of this last case also suggests a need for curative and regulatory care and health promotion.

None of the cases in this chapter deals with a multiperson unit (family, group/aggregate, or community) as patient. However, the reader can further challenge himself/herself by applying the nursing process to the "patient" identified and assessed in Exercise: Basic Conditioning Factors of Groups/Communities in Chapter 3 (see p. 33). This exercise asks the reader to assess the basic conditioning factors of a multiperson unit. Further tasks in step I of the nursing process require that the nurse make nursing decisions about the needs for self-care and dependent care in the multiperson unit (therapeutic self-care demand) and the abilities of the multiperson unit to meet those needs (care agency); judgments about the relationship between therapeutic self-care demand and care agency will lead to conclusions about the need for nursing care (based on identifications of care deficits). Apply step II of the nursing process to design appropriate nursing systems and formulate plan(s) of care to address the prioritized care deficits of the multiperson unit as patient. Discuss issues of regulation and control as part of step III of the nursing process.

Glossary

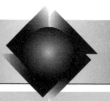

ability   the capacity, power, or potential of being able to act.

act   that which is the thing done; a deed performed by a person.

action   an activity; an act as carried out or performed.

action demand   the action or set of actions necessary to meet a self-care requisite; a component part of therapeutic self-care demand.

action limitations   restrictions or limitations in a person's abilities for producing action that prohibits or inhibits the performance of action (self-care action, dependent care action, or nursing action); types of action limitations are (1) limitations of knowing, (2) limitations of judging and decision-making, and (3) limitations for engagement in result-achieving action.

action repertoire   a series or set of sequential or related discrete actions necessary to accomplish expected results.

action sequence   a chronological series of ordered, consecutive discrete actions.

action system   an organized series of actions clustered or sequenced to occur together for the purpose of achieving foreseen results.

adequacy   a term applied to a judgment of self-care (or dependent care) agency identifying whether the abilities of agency are sufficient to perform those actions necessary to achieve therapeutic self-care (or dependent care); may also apply to a judgment about nursing agency identifying whether the abilities are sufficient to perform the required nursing care.

agency   ability, power, capability. In self-care deficit theory of nursing (SCDTN) the abilities that comprise agency may be those of the self-care agent, dependent care agent, or nurse agent.

agent   the performer of action, the person taking action or responsible for action. In self-care deficit theory of nursing (SCDTN) the following are agents: self-care agent, dependent care agent, or nurse agent.

basic conditioning factors (BCFs)   fundamental characteristics common to all persons that identify and contribute to the uniqueness of each person, the person's situation, and the abilities of an individual to carry out self-care or dependent care. There are 10 basic conditioning factors that condition/modify the self-care (or dependent care) agent, therapeutic self-care demand, self-care (or dependent care) agency, and nursing agency: (1) age, (2) gender, (3) developmental state, (4) health state, (5) health care system, (6) sociocultural/spiritual orientation, (7) family system, (8) patterns of living, (9) environment, and (10) available resources.

care measure   term synonymous with care action, whether self-care (or dependent care) action or nursing action.

care production the process of producing care (self-care, dependent care, or nursing care) through the execution, regulation, and control of planned care actions.

deliberate action purposeful, goal-seeking activity in which the goal sought is known before engaging in chosen activities leading to goal attainment. Consists of two problem-solving phases: (1) estimative and transitional operations leading to choice of action(s) to be taken and (2) productive operations resulting in implementation of chosen action(s).

demand for dependent care the amount and type of dependent care that the dependent care agent must provide to meet some or all of the self-care requisites of the dependent care recipient, largely determined by the self-care deficits of the dependent care recipient.

dependent care the production and practice of activities directed toward another's self-care requisites to regulate that person's own functioning, thus maintaining life, health, and well-being of that person.

dependent care action care measure(s) carried out or performed by a person providing dependent care (dependent care agent) with the intent of meeting self-care requisites of the person receiving dependent care (dependent care recipient).

dependent care agency (DCA) the abilities of the dependent care agent; the abilities of the person who performs activities on behalf of another person (dependent care recipient) aimed at meeting that person's self-care requisites; the abilities to care for another.

dependent care agent the person who performs care actions on behalf of another person (the dependent care recipient); the person who provides and performs dependent care.

dependent care deficit (DCD) the deficit relationship that exists when the *combined* agency of the dependent care recipient and the dependent care agent are insufficient for meeting the therapeutic self-care demands of the dependent care recipient.

$$[\text{TSCD (of DCR)} > \text{SCA (of DCR)} + \text{DCA} = \text{DCD}]$$

dependent care dyad/unit the two (dyad) or more (unit) persons who are active participants in the dependent care system, including one dependent care recipient and one or more dependent care agents; successful interaction and working of these persons as a unit is essential for success of the dependent care system.

dependent care limitations restrictions or limitations in dependent care agency that prohibit or inhibit the performance of dependent care actions; deficiencies in dependent care agency that lead to dependent care deficits; three types of limitations are (1) limitations of knowing, (2) limitations of judging and decision-making, and (3) limitations for engagement in result-achieving action.

dependent care system an action system designed, created, and produced for the provision of dependent care; synonymous with dependent care.

dependent care recipient (DCR) the person in need of and receiving dependent care provided by another.

desired outcome an outcome that is valued above others, that is, the one wanted most.

developmental needs in self-care those needs for self-care that pertain to the control or management of conditions or resources necessary to support or promote normal human development.

developmental self-care requisites (DSCRs) the category of self-care requisites derived from and associated with human development. There are two types: (1) those arising from conditions and events that normally occur at stages in the life cycle (i.e., maturational) and (2) those arising from specific conditions and events that may adversely affect development (i.e., situational).

estimative operation investigative and reflective actions that are part of the intentional phase of deliberate action and seek to discover what is and what should be.

existing self–care deficit a self-care deficit in which the current self-care abilities (agency) are inadequate for meeting the current self-care requisites.

expected outcome an outcome that is anticipated via a process of investigation and selection; the selected outcome that should occur following given actions.

goal of nursing according to the self-care deficit theory of nursing, the ultimate purpose of nursing care is to ensure the achievement/accomplishment of therapeutic self-care (dependent care).

habits for self–care action(s) for self-care that, through frequent repetition, become a routinized part of a person's usual behavior; self-care actions performed so routinely that they are done almost without conscious awareness (particularly of the estimative and transitional self-care operations).

health care system the total complex of related and available services for health promotion and prevention, regulation, stabilization, or remediation of health deviations in an array of settings (i.e., in institutionalized agencies such as hospitals, public or private clinics, long-term care facilities, and preferred provider or health maintenance organizations) and provided by an array of health care providers; the totality of service-oriented action systems of health care providers (i.e., traditional health care providers [e.g., nursing, medicine, physical therapy, occupational therapy, respiratory therapy, speech and hearing therapies] and nontraditional health care providers [e.g., herbalist or shaman]); factors that arise from the health care system

serve as basic conditioning factors.

health deviation illness or injury, either physical or mental, that results in (1) pathology, defects, or disabilities, (2) alterations in physical structure or function, or (3) alterations in required and normal patterns of self-care (or dependent care).

health deviation self–care requisites (HDSCRs) the category of self-care requisites that arise from (1) genetic and constitutional defects, (2) human structural and functional deviations, and (3) the effects of medical diagnostic and treatment measures. Impact on universal and developmental self-care requisites must be considered. (NOTE: Health deviation self-care requisites are derived from physical or mental health deviations.)

health focus (or health care focus) a classification of the central issues of health care that suggests the types of health care goals, the kinds of health care required (including nursing), and any existing or projected obstacles to self-care (dependent care) using the following criteria: presence or absence of health deviation(s), the overall general quality of health state or values assigned to health state, and the life-cycle events and conditions related to existing or projected health care needs.

health state a compilation of the assessed structural, physical, functional, and mental integrity of a person and judgments of the relationship of the assessed data with norms established for persons of a similar age, gender, or developmental stage; also includes the person's own perception of his or her status; factors from the health state serve as basic conditioning factors.

human capabilities and dispositions abilities and inclinations of humans that are foundational to all forms of action, including (but not limited to) self-care, dependent care, and nursing care.

human foundational abilities abilities of humans that are the basis for development or exercise of more specialized abilities associated with the estimative, transitional, and productive abilities associated with the estimative, transitional, and productive operations of deliberate action; part of or synonymous with human capabilities and dispositions.

knowledge repertoire those cognitive and intellectual abilities of agency (self-care agency, dependent care agency, or nursing agency) that enable a person to inquire, learn, retain, reason, and make decisions and that contribute to the abilities for valuing, prioritizing, and perservering.

legitimate patient of nursing the patient evidencing health-related or health-derived existing or projected self-care deficits, thus having a need for nursing care; the patient may be an individual person, a dependent care dyad/unit, a family, a group or aggregate, or a community.

methods of helping methods used by nurses in helping patients overcome self-care limitations that lead to existing or projected self-care deficits or dependent care limitations that lead to existing or projected dependent care deficits. There are five general methods of helping: (1) acting or doing for another, (2) guiding another, (3) supporting another, (4) providing a developmental environment, and (5) teaching another.

multiperson unit a grouping of two or more persons with some relationship forming a social unit (e.g., a family, a group or aggregate, or a community) in which the unit is viewed as a single whole entity.

nurse agent the *person* who performs nursing care; one prepared through specialized nursing education to provide nursing care; synonymous with nurse.

nursing actions actions selected, performed, and executed by nurses via exercise of nursing agency for the prescription, planning, and production of nursing; includes those associated with the social, interpersonal, and professional-technological components of the process of nursing.

nursing agency specialized abilities of nurses for performing forms of deliberate action used to assist patients in overcoming or compensating for health-derived or health-related self-care deficits; abilities learned through nursing education and experience and conditioned or modified by the basic conditioning factors; specialized abilities employed by nurses to determine the need for, the design of, and the production of nursing care for persons in a wide variety of nursing situations.

nursing care a specialized form of health care generated and performed by nurses (i.e., nurse agents) that addresses actual or potential problems posed by health-derived and health-related existing or projected self-care (or dependent care) deficits, with the intent of ensuring the accomplishment of therapeutic self-care (or dependent care); the care system produced by nurses exercising nursing agency for patients with existing or projected self-care (or dependent care) deficits.

nursing diagnosis statement a statement that expresses the patient's existing or projected problem areas that can and should be addressed by nursing; for self-care deficit theory of nursing, an expression of the patient's existing or projected self-care (or dependent care) deficits.

nursing knowledge the practical and applied fields of knowledge of and about nursing and their related modes of inquiry and methods of understanding; knowledge that enables nurses to engage in and produce nursing; in relation to self-care deficit theory of nursing, the following are identified as the seven fields of nursing knowledge: nursing social field, nursing as a profession and occupation, nursing jurisprudence, nursing history, nursing ethics, nursing science, and nursing economics.

nursing practice engagement in and responsibility for the prescription, planning, production, and provision of nursing care to patients (singly or in multiperson units) to bring about outcomes related to the health or well-being of the patient; activities of nurses producing nursing care during periods of contact with patients.

nursing process the conscious, systematic method of problem-solving and decision-making that, combined with applied knowledge, enables nurses to select and perform nursing actions that (1) establish nursing relationships with legitimate patients, (2) provide the type and amount of nursing care required by the patient, and (3) judge the effectiveness of the nursing care provided and the need for changes in that care; in association with self-care deficit theory of nursing, the orderly steps of diagnosis and prescription, design and planning, and regulation and control.

nursing relationship the interactive association or partnership between nurse and patient for the purpose of the provision of nursing care.

nursing situation points in time or place in which nurses interact with persons with health-derived or health-related self-care or dependent care deficits for the purpose of producing and providing nursing care.

nursing system the series of organized, concrete actions performed by nurses in collaboration with the patients; an interlocking system of actions representing all the actions and interactions of the nurse and patient in a nursing situation; three components of the process of nursing (the social, interpersonal, and professional-technological) exist concurrently for the delivery of nursing care in nursing situations. There are three types of nursing systems: (1) wholly compensatory, (2) partly compensatory, and (3) supportive-educative.

operability a term for a judgment about self-care (or dependent care) agency identifying whether present abilities can be, should be, or are being exercised (i.e., if the use of abilities is both wise and safe); may also apply to nursing agency, identifying whether a nurse's abilities can be, should be, or are being exercised in the production of nursing care.

operation an intellectual or psychomotor action directed toward a goal or end result.

outcome the end or final result(s) toward which action is directed.

particularized self-care requisites (PSCRs) statements or expressions of self-care requisites formulated to provide specific, individual qualifications about the need for self-care and the ways and means (actions) necessary to meet that need; action-oriented statements that specify the degree and type of actions necessary to meet a self-care requisite.

partly compensatory nursing system the type of nursing system in which both the nurse and the patient engage in care actions aimed at the accomplishment of therapeutic self-care. The nurse assists with or performs those actions for those self-care requisites that the patient cannot or should not perform, while the patient performs all other self-care (or dependent care) actions.

plan of care the organized set of actions selected for the purpose of accomplishing a desired end result; in self-care (or dependent care) the set of organized, selected self-care (or dependent care) actions intended to meet the self-care requisites and accomplish self-care (dependent care); in nursing the set of organized, selected helping actions (derived from the methods of helping) and role prescriptions intended to address problems posed by existing or projected self-care (or dependent care) deficits and ensure the accomplishment of therapeutic self-care (or dependent care).

power components a set of defined powers within agency that enable the exercise of abilities related to the self-care operations (estimative, transitional, and productive) of the intentional and productive phases of deliberate action.

process a series or set of related activities that lead to or are directed toward a particular result.

process of nursing the combined social, interpersonal, and professional-technological components of the practice of nursing that, when occurring simultaneously, result in nursing practice.

productive operation psychomotor and intellectual actions that make up the productive phase of deliberate action and seek to produce intended actions for meeting expected outcomes and validate effectiveness in doing so.

projected self-care deficit a self-care deficit in which the self-care abilities (agency) are inadequate for meeting self-care requisites reasonably and logically anticipated in the near future.

repertoire sets or clusters of related processes or skills.

requisite a need for care and the actions necessary to meet that need.

role prescription the process of ascribing and assigning roles and the tasks assigned to those roles.

self-care the production and practice of actions directed toward one's self or one's environment to regulate one's own functioning, thus achieving and maintaining life, health, and well-being; self-care actions are learned over time in the sociocultural and family context of the individual.

self-care action care measure carried out or performed by a person providing self-care (self-care agent) with the intent of meeting his or her own self-care requisites.

self-care agency (SCA) the complex set of abilities of an individual to engage in or perform self-care; such abilities are culturally derived and learned and developed over time.

self-care agent the person engaged in the performance of self-care and performing those actions for one's self.

self-care deficit (SCD) the deficit relationship that exists when the demand for therapeutic self-care exceeds the person's ability to perform self-care (self-care agency). TSCD > SCA = SCD

self-care limitations restrictions or limitations in self-care agency that prohibit or inhibit the performance of self-care actions; deficiencies in self-care agency that lead to self-care deficits; three types of self-care limitations are (1) limitations of knowing, (2) limitations of judging and decision-making, and (3) limitations for engagement in result-achieving action.

self-care operation intellectual, valuing, and psychomotor processes associated with deliberate action directed toward self-care; therefore self-care operations are estimative, transitional, or productive operations directed toward the purpose of accomplishing the deliberate action of self-care.

self-care requisites (SCRs) the needs for self-care and the related care actions necessary for achieving or maintaining life, structural and functional integrity, health, and well-being; there are three types or categories: (1) universal, (2) developmental, and (3) health deviation; the purposes for self-care.

self-care system an action system designed, created, and produced for the provision of self-care; synonymous with self-care.

sets of operations clusters of related operations (i.e., actions) that may or may not be sequential and that delineate the ways and means of achieving a specific result.

skill repertoire sets of cognitive, perceptual, manipulative, communicative, and interpersonal abilities of agency (self-care agency, dependent care agency, and nursing agency) that enable a person in performance of actions requiring physical movement and manipulation.

supportive educative nursing system the type of nursing system in which the patient can and should perform all the actions for self-care (or dependent care) but can only do so after learning what to do or how to perform the required self-care (or dependent care) actions (i.e., the patient must develop further self-care [or dependent care] abilities) or after having adequate support to carry out these actions.

technologies the knowledge and related intellectual and psychomotor skills essential to the action.

therapeutic self-care demand (TSCD) the *totality* of self-care actions to be performed for some duration of time to meet self-care requisites (action demands) using valid methods and related sets of operations; the total set of action demands for any given point of time necessary to achieve optimal health and well-being.

USCR + DSCR + HDSCR = TSCD

transitional operation judging and decision-making actions that are part of the intentional phase of deliberate action; are preceded by estimative operations, and seek to make choices about the desirability of expected outcomes and what to do to achieve the outcome.

universal self-care requisites (USCRs) the category of self-care requisites that are basic and common to all humans and are constantly present; these needs must be met to achieve optimal health and well-being. There are eight universal self-care requisites: (1) air, (2) food, (3) water, (4) elimination, (5) activity and rest, (6) solitude and social interaction, (7) prevention of hazards, and (8) normalcy.

wholly compensatory nursing system the type of nursing system in which the nurse compensates for the patient's inability to engage in any self-care by performing actions necessary to meet self-care requisites. The three subtypes of wholly compensatory nursing systems are designed for the following: (1) those persons unable to perform any deliberate action; (2) those persons who can not or should not perform deliberate actions even though they may be able to think, decide, and judge data; and (3) those persons who are unable to make reasoned judgments and decisions even though they may be able to physically perform actions.

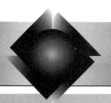

Bibliography

American Nurses Association. (1980). *Nursing: A social policy statement* (Publication No. NP-6335M). Kansas City, MO: Author.

Backscheider, J. E. (1974). Self-care requisites, self-care capabilities and nursing systems in the diabetic nurse management clinic. *American Journal of Public Health, 64,* 1138-1146.

Blegen, M. A., & Tripp-Reimer, T. (1994). The nursing theory-nursing research connection. In J. McCloskey & H. K. Grace (Eds.), *Current issues in nursing* (4th ed., pp. 87-91). St. Louis, MO: Mosby.

Burns, N., & Grove, S. K. (1993). *The practice of nursing research* (2nd ed.). Philadelphia: Saunders.

Christ, M. A., & Hohloch, F. J. (1988). *Gerontologic nursing: A study and learning tool.* Springhouse, PA: Springhouse.

Christensen, P. J., & Kenney, J. W. (1995). *Nursing process: Application of conceptual models* (4th ed.). St. Louis, MO: Mosby.

Conant, L. H. (1992). Closing the practice-theory gap. In L. H. Nicholl (Ed.), *Perspectives on nursing theory* (2nd ed, pp. 461-462). Philadelphia: Lippincott.

Firlit, S. L. (1994). The nursing theory—nursing practice connection. In J. McCloskey & H. K. Grace (Eds.), *Current issues in nursing* (4th ed, pp. 76-81). St. Louis, MO: Mosby.

Keck, J. F. (1994). Terminology of theory development. In A. Marriner-Tomey (Ed.), *Nursing theorists and their work* (3rd ed., pp. 17-26). St. Louis, MO: Mosby.

Maas, M., Buckwalter, K. C., & Hardy, M. (1991). *Nursing diagnoses and interventions for the elderly.* Redwood City, CA: Addison-Wesley Nursing.

Marriner-Tomey, A. (1994). Introduction to analysis of nursing theories. In A. Marriner-Tomey (Ed.), *Nursing theorists and their work* (3rd ed, pp. 3-16). St. Louis, MO: Mosby.

Meleis, A. I. (1991). *Theoretical nursing: Development and progress* (2nd ed.). Philadelphia: Lippincott.

Murray, R. B., & Zentner, J. P (1993). *Nursing assessment and health promotion: Strategies through the life span* (5th ed.). Norwalk, CT: Appleton & Lange.

Nicholl, L. H. (1992). Nursing theory and practice. In L. H. Nicholl (Ed.), *Perspectives on nursing theory* (2nd ed., pp. 461-462). Philadelphia: Lippincott.

Orem, D. (1995). *Nursing: Concepts of practice* (5th ed.). St. Louis, MO: Mosby.

Orem, D. (1991). *Nursing: Concepts of practice* (4th ed.). St. Louis, MO: Mosby.

Orem, D. (1985). *Nursing: Concepts of practice* (3rd ed.). St. Louis, MO: Mosby.

Orem, D. (Ed.). (1979). *Concept formalization in nursing: Process and product* (2nd ed.). Boston, MA: Little, Brown & Company.

Wong, D. L. (1995). *Whaley & Wong's nursing care of infants and children* (5th ed.). St. Louis, MO: Mosby.

Yura, H., & Walsh, M. (1988). *The nursing process: Assessing, planning, implementing, and evaluating* (5th ed.). Norwalk, CT: Appleton & Lange.

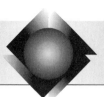

INDEX

Dependent care system, 10
Design and plan step
case studies in, 123, 124
in nursing process, 113-115
Developmental defects, nursing systems and, 93
Developmental environment, providing, methods of helping and, 91
Developmental self-care requisites (DSCRs), 9, 42, 46-52, 62
maturation and, 51
situational impact on, 53
types of, 47-52
Developmental state
basic conditioning factors and, 24, 26, 28, 32
in case studies, 125, 129, 133
Diagnosis and prescription step
case studies in, 120-123
in nursing process, 106-112, 113
Diagnostic statements, nursing, formulation of, 112, 113
Dispositions, human, self-care agency and, 66
Doing for another, methods of helping and, 90
DSCRs; *see* Developmental self-care requisites

E

Elimination, universal self-care requisites and, 43, 44, 45, 46
Environment
basic conditioning factors and, 25, 27, 31, 32
in case studies, 128, 131-132, 136
Estimative self-care operations, 21, 23, 65, 73, 110-111
Existing self-care deficit, 13, 72

F

Factor
basic conditioning; *see* Basic conditioning factors
definition of, 24
Family members, 86
Family system
basic conditioning factors and, 25, 27, 28, 32
in case studies, 127, 131, 135
Foundational concepts of self-care deficit theory of nursing, 19-33
Functioning, integrated, stabilization of, nursing systems and, 94

G

Gender, basic conditioning factors and, 24, 26, 30, 32
Generic approach to nursing process, 105, 106
Genetic defects, nursing systems and, 93
Grand theory, 2
Groups, basic conditioning factors of, 33
Guiding another, methods of helping and, 90

H

Hazards, prevention of, universal self-care requisites and, 44, 46
HDSCRs; *see* Health deviation self-care requisites

Self-care—cont'd
  responsibility of, 39
  as right, 39
  self-care agency and, 65
  sequence and, 39
  voluntary, 39
Self-care agency (SCA), 11, 13, 25, 64-71, 80, 81-82, 84-85, 86
  assessment of, 71, 109-112
  content of, 109
  versus dependent care agency, 79-80
  form and content of, 65-71, 109
  nursing agency versus, 85
  self-care limitations within, 69-70
  therapeutic self-care demand and, 72
Self-care agent, 36, 81, 108-109
Self-care deficit (SCD), 12, 35-82, 72, 75
  complete, 74, 75
  determination of, in nursing process, 112
  existing, 13, 72
  partial, 74, 75
  projected, 13, 73
  theory of, 6, 7, 11-14, 71-75
Self-care deficit theory of nursing (SCDTN), 2, 4, 6
  articulations among self-care requisites in, 56-58
  case studies in, 119-137
  composite particularized self-care requisite statements in, 58-61
  conceptual framework for, 96
  deliberate action in, 20-23
  dependent care in, 76-80
  developmental self-care requisites in, 46-52
  foundational concepts of, 19-33
  health deviation self-care requisites in, 52-56
  key concepts of, 35-82
  overview of, 5-18
  self-care in, 36-39, 40-41
  self-care agency in, 64-71
  self-care deficit in, 71-75
  self-care requisites in, 39-61
  self-care/dependent care in, 6-11, 76-80
  supporting background of, 6-7
  theory of nursing system, 6, 7, 14-15
  theory of self-care deficit, 6, 7, 11-14, 71-75
  theory of self-care/dependent care, 6-11, 76-80
  therapeutic self-care demands in, 61-64
  universal self-care requisites in, 43-46
Self-care demand, therapeutic, calculation of, in nursing process, 109
Self-care limitations, 12
  self-care agency and, 69-70, 74
Self-care requisite statements, particularized, 58-61
Self-care requisites (SCRs), 9, 11, 16, 24, 39-61, 59
  articulations among, 56-58